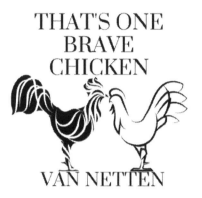

COVID-19 CHICKEN AND A MIRACLE

STEADY AS WE GO

That Is One Brave Chicken!

Sarah VanNetten

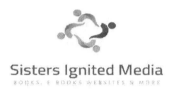

Sisters Ignited Media
BOOKS, E BOOKS WEBSITES & MORE

DISCLAIMER

Find us at: www.SIMPInc.info/

Copyright 2021 – Sisters Ignited Media and Publishing Inc. / Sarah VanNetten

All rights to this book are reserved. No permission is given for any part of this book to be reproduced, transmitted in any form, or means; electronic or mechanical, stored in a retrieval system, photocopied, recorded, scanned, or otherwise. Any of these actions require the proper written permission of the author.

Sisters Ignited Media and Publishing Inc.

First Printing Edition, 2021
ISBN: 9798475414200

DEDICATION:

To my husband, Mike, Mikey, your Chicken, to our children Zack, Alexis, Ryan, and Holly. To our community of friends, health care workers, Covid patients and their families. To prayer warriors near and far, and to the One Almighty. I dedicate the story of our journey.

Love Sarah

INTRODUCTION:

On April 8th of 2021 Mike VanNetten, a 45- year-old chicken farmer, husband, and father of four from Norfolk County, Ontario went to the local hospital with difficulty breathing. This book tells the story through his wife's eyes of the first 46 days of his journey with Covid 19.

The devotions that you are about to read are inspired by Sarah's daily words, her faith, and her courage. Sarah's daily posts on social media exploded to thousands of people across the country following their story.

There is more than a great story in this book, there is a divine sense of purpose as you read through each day, you will feel the strength and spiritual growth that Sarah experiences and shares. She doesn't hold back on the bad days, and she always celebrates her life with Mike. You will grow with her through their incredible story.

It is our hope that this story educates its readers about the reality of COVID 19 and what it does to the human body. From, Mike's medically induced coma to helping Mike to know and understand the faith journey of the days he missed and how the community, friends, family, and the medical teams, rallied around them to show their love and support for him and his family.

The VanNetten journey will resonate with and help other families going through similar situations with a way to connect emotionally and spiritually. Along with anyone who has suffered from prayed for or stood at the bedside of an ill loved one.

But most importantly this story will guide you and anyone who reads it. It will show others how strong God is and the power of prayer. The importance of a relationship with God and that, miracles do still happen when God is invited in.

Everyone needs a prayer warrior, maybe you are that warrior for someone?

Contents

Dedication:	*iii*
Introduction:	*iv*
The journey begins	*1*
God has a Plan	*3*
__HELP	6
Lights for Chicken	*8*
With you, always	*10*
God's Love Saturates Us.	*13*
Hold One's Own	*15*
"Steady as We Go."	*18*
HOPE	20
BATTLE	25
WAIT	29
God Provides	*32*
BELIEVE	35
COURAGE	39
BREATHE	45
GRACE	49
GOOD FATHER	57
YOU NEVER LET GO	62
"I NEED YOU"	*67*
Strength	*72*
Hallelujah	*75*
Comfort	*80*
Just Be Held	*84*

CORNERSTONE	88
WHILE I WAIT	93
PRAY	98
CALM	103
Breathe -Take 2	107
RESCUE	112
POWERFUL	119
LOVE	124
PEACE	129
RESILIENCE and PERSEVERANCE	134
BLESSED	138
Oh, My Heart…	143
TRANSFORMATION	149
STEADY AS WE GO	155
THERE is NO ME, WITHOUT YOU.	161
MIRACLE	166
We all have mountains	171
Don't Gamble with Your Faith!	175
Baby Steps	181
Proud of Mike	186
Detours	191
Keep Looking Forward	197
Lean on Me	202
You Must Believe	207
Ginger ale	213
CHA, CHA	218
Stay Grounded	223
No do overs	229
The Lessons of Pain	238
Patience for Patients	243

Moving on Up	249
Lazy Saturday	254
Steady Sunday	258
Give it to God	263
The Gout	268
The Little Things	274
Good Days	278
Beautiful Days	282
Purpose	287
Another Chapter Closes	291
Rehab!	296
I PROMISE TO CATCH YOU!	301
Keeping on Track	306
Entering the Seventies	310
Keep your Focus	314
Golden Days	318
Father's Day	322
Find your Contentment	327
Adversity	336
We are all in the same Boat	340
Enjoy your Tuesday!	346
I Wanted to tell you a little secret	355
A little Note, before you go.	358
A few photos from our journey:	360

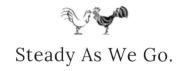

Steady As We Go.

THE JOURNEY BEGINS

Day 1 /April 8th

Tonight, I write a post, not as someone who is choosing a side or picking a government or a right or wrong … I do know one thing. Covid is real, it's not a government trying to screw its people, it's politicians trying to make choices in a world where they cannot win. It's … I think I have a cold… I will be ok, too suddenly, I'm not ok.

People, friends, take it seriously… for the love of God stay at home. This is life. Pray to the only God who can get us out of this. Pray for my Mike, pray for your neighbour, your enemy, your anybody.

COVID is real. Think otherwise and join my sadness. Stay home… keep businesses closed … 'be still and let God'. Our only hope.

Love Sarah

Scripture: Psalm 46:10

[10] He says, "Be still, and know that I am God;
   I will be exalted among the nations, I will be exalted in the earth."

Reflection:

Isn't it wonderful that a God so powerful can create a universe with a word, ask us to be quiet and still so that we can hear Him? It is in those still moments, in the weakness of our hearts that we hear our God.

Take the time to clear away the distractions of your world so that you can hear your mighty God, whisper to your soul.

"Be still and know that the Lord is in control. I won't be afraid. You are here. You silence all my fear."

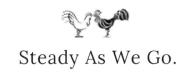

Steady As We Go.

GOD HAS A PLAN

Day 2 / April 9th

I wanted to thank everyone for the overwhelming love, kindness, prayers, and concern for Mike. I never expected the support I would receive over posting about Mike... but I am so glad I did.

He needs to be thought of often right now and prayed for and have lots of love and energy sent in his way. He deserves it and he needs it.

For all those wondering. This is what I know and have learned. Mike is in Burlington in ICU. He has been officially diagnosed with COVID-19.

This afternoon I received a call from Burlington ...it was a social worker who was in with Mike (I wish I caught her name; she is praiseworthy). She realizes it is hard to be away from loved ones and you can't picture where they are, so she painted me a picture and this is what it looks like. Mike is in a large private room with a private bathroom. He has a big window with a beautiful view of Lake Ontario and a rock garden outside his window as well. He has a big screen tv and a chair to sit on if he can. She wanted us to know he is comfortable. He can be always seen by nurses. She could not give me medical information, but she could give me peace of mind and knowing he is being cared for. Mike was sitting in his chair with her, and I spoke with him for one moment. I told him how loved he is and how many great friends and family he has. I did not take long... you can tell how hard it is for him to breathe and talk but he knows how much love there is for him and how missed he is. He did tell me that he will be home in no time... and I will hold him to it.

Before supper I called his nurse for today, Carolina, to see how he is, and this is what I learned. She was quite easy to talk to and very caring. She said Mike kept apologizing for having to trouble her (or maybe using the moves that we all know only Mike has). He is very dependent on oxygen... as my smarter friends explained to me. Mike is on 70 percent oxygen. When you and I breathe, only 21 percent of that breath is oxygen. That is usually all we need. This means Mike is requiring 70 percent (instead of 21) to be sure his blood delivers enough oxygen to his brain and vital organs (thank you Rob Preston for the explanation).

He no longer has a fever, and he is on the Covid drugs. Carolina said she is hoping he is headed in the right direction. Things can change quickly, but she is hopeful.

I can't say enough about these workers... Norfolk General Hospital, where he started his care, to the fast-acting doctors... to Angie Miller who took care of Mike. You were what he needed. It meant everything.

Now to Joseph Brant in Burlington. These workers really are the superheroes... they deserve our admiration and love and I think they want to go home, so friends do what we can... stay home, stay safe, love your family, be kind and always keep praying.

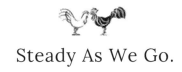

Steady As We Go.

There is power in prayer and although I'm not always sure of it, God has a plan and in his eyes it's all under control.

love Sarah

Scripture: Proverbs 19:21 "Many are the plans in a man's heart, but it is the Lord's purpose that prevails."

Reflection:

The best way to have our lives go as planned, is to align our plans with God's.

We may not always understand the why of His work, but we can take solace in knowing that God is good, and all things will be used for His glory.

God wastes nothing, not even our sorrows. There is a purpose for every moment of our lives.

HELP

Day 3/ April 10th

How do I even say this...? I just want all those who have been following and asking about Mike, to know that they put him on a vent today.

His body needs the help and the rest. I am not expecting a response... save your typing, send your thoughts and prayers to God. Send your positive energy to my most favorite person in the world... My Mikey, your Chicken, my kid's dad, a son, a brother, and the best friend many of us have ever had the privilege to know.

I spoke to him. He knows he is loved... that all of us are ok at home. He has countless friends. We need him. He's coming back to us. Prayer and positive thoughts only! Mike has this.

Love Sarah

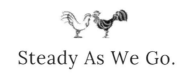

Steady As We Go.

Scripture:

Psalms 46:1
God is our refuge and strength, a very present help in trouble.

Reflection:

     He will not leave you or forsake you. God is a loving Father; He is ever present in the good times and the terrible. Sometimes we need more help than what the people in our lives can give.

     Only God can help in these times. Lean on Him. He wants his kids to reach out to him. Let Him be there for you in all your times, both good and bad.

Author Sarah VanNetten

LIGHTS FOR CHICKEN

Day 4 / April 11th

I spoke to Mike's nurse. Today's nurse's name is Kristen. Mike had a good night. He went down on his oxygen a bit which is good... I did not ask the number. I can't get caught up in numbers right now. Down is good that's all that matters right now. He is still on his stomach; they are flipping him at 10:00. His doctor has not been in yet but I'm sure he will call after he is.

Kristen will call me sometime today before she goes to see him in his room, and I will talk to Mike.

Our friend Guy, who lives down the road from the hospital is walking there everyday to touch the wall and let Mike know to stay strong. He has this and God has him.

Facebook Message from a friend: Our buddy, our friend, our amazing Chicken Man needs our support!!!

There is no more selfless man among us!!! His wit, sense of humour, love for his family, and zest for life has touched us all at least once somewhere along the way!!! I know you all have been praying for him and I know he feels the love that surrounds him!!!!

Let's show Mike our love just a little more.

Find a way to light up your porch, your garage, your roof, your anything!!!

Let's leave a light on for Chicken.

He will be home soon!!!

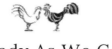

Steady As We Go.

Send me a pic of your creation and I will put together a "scrapbook" for his return home!!!

Please share this with as many people as you know!!! There is no such thing as too much love for the VanNetten family!!!

Please be safe and pray for our dearest Chicken!!!

You know we all want to hear his smart-ass comments when this is all over!!

Thanks, Dovey.

Scripture:

Isaiah 43:2 "When you go through deep waters, I will be with you."

Reflection: God never stops working. He is working on Mike at this moment. He is a miracle worker, a promise keeper our light in the darkness. He wants you to ask for Him. He is both willing and able. You are never alone. You are highly favoured. Reach out and God promises that He is there.

Author Sarah VanNetten

WITH YOU, ALWAYS

Day 5 / April 12th

To say that I am overwhelmed would be an understatement. I am scared beyond anything I could ever have imagined... yet I have this amazing thing that has happened around us.

First off, an update on Mike. He is doing ok... to sum it all up today for the most part has been a good day! His turn from his tummy to his back this morning was far easier on his body than yesterday. His oxygen levels rebounded quicker and Kristen (Mike's nurse) and Dr. Schkitt, were pleased.

The Dr was my first call this morning and the most important thing that I took away is not to overreact. We are going to have some good things happen and some bad things, remain calm, don't get caught up. All his numbers were within a range of where they should be.

I called Kristen at noon for an update to see how Mike is and to ask to have the phone put to his ear again today. She suggested I Facetime him.

To which I thought, I can't, I'm not strong enough but if Mike is strong enough than so am I. So, as I prepared for this, Kristen also said that they had taken him a wee bit off his paralyzer drugs, and he responded well. He had his eyes open, and she told him I would be calling soon, and he attempted a thumbs up (He hears her).

It was difficult and painful, but he looked like my Mikey. I had a beer with him (liquid courage). These are a few things I told him. Firstly, that he slept through his most

Steady As We Go.

favorite day of the year, NHL trade deadline day, I told him what the Leafs, had done and that the parade is fast approaching. I told him the farm is fine, we have it. I told him that our friend, Guy is sitting outside the hospital every day talking to him (hoping that he doesn't get admitted for being that crazy guy). And I told him about all of you.... that people, some of you who I don't even know have shown this man the most incredible support that I have ever been privy to witness. I am astounded. I shouldn't be amazed. Mike has always surrounded him with the best of the best. "The Lights on for Chicken campaign makes me cry. I am thankful for you, one and all.

I can never express what this means to me and to our kids. Small communities, we have each other.

One last thing while talking to Mike today- he did try to open his eyes, but it was effort, I told him to close them to rest and his only job is oxygen levels. Kevin got to visit him tonight! I'm so grateful. I want it to be me but for now Mike is learning all about buy and sell prices of seed and cropping but he is also knowing how loved he is and all about his friends and family. I know this is a long one. No individual texts tonight. We love you all with our whole hearts. Tomorrow I am sending some pics to his nurse to print for his room. She also said I can send sayings, quotes, whatever. Nothing makes Mike happier than The Gambler. So that's what I have decided for words to be written. Kenny Rogers.

Keep Praying, light up the night. You have this my Mikey!

Love Sarah

Scripture:

Matthew 28:20 "I am with you always"

Reflection:

It is not until our life is shaken off it's axis that we realize the world does not revolve around us. It is when we are plucked out of our normal lives, that we realize that we were created for something more. We are here to love and be loved. We are here to share, God and receive God. We are here to lift one another up. Our true joy is not hidden in the obscure; it is all around us in every part of the gift called life.

Seek God first and you will find the joy in all things.

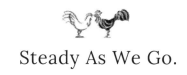

Steady As We Go.

GOD'S LOVE SATURATES US.

Day 6 /April 13th

Mike was airlifted from Burlington to Hamilton today. My update tonight … Mike made it to the General. He has received the ECMO surgery. His oxygen is good. They will be doing constant blood work. The surgery took about an hour. He is on his back now, but they can prone him if need be. His nurse tonight is Marjory, but I spoke with Nadia. … beautiful, calming. His saturation is greater than 90…. which is fantastic … they accept 85, so he is doing better. I will call anytime throughout night for an update. Nadia ensured me there are so many doctors up on his floor, always. They are working tirelessly for Mike and all those suffering.

I can't explain my emotions… I can't express my love for my friends. I love you all.

Quote:

"Be still… I am fighting your battles"

God

#Leavealightonforchicken
#Mikeysgotvthis

Scripture:

Deuteronomy 20:4

"For the Lord, your God is he who goes with you to fight for you against your enemies, to give you the victory."

Reflection:

There are times when it is obvious that things are not within our control. The truth is things rarely are. Life happens. We have no control over random illness, accidents, the way others treat us. There is only one thing that we can control. We can control our response to what is happening in our lives. We choose our reactions. We choose how to carry on.

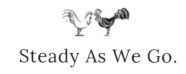

Steady As We Go.

HOLD ONE'S OWN

Day 7 /April 14th

First off … why does Facebook ask: "What is on your mind?"… possibly the stupidest question ever.

I think everyone knows what is on my mind, it is on everyone's … it is the constant thought, emotion, prayer, memory, thought, all mind consuming, it's Mike. This is getting harder. I will not lie. I only want to update with "ups."

Let me tell you what I know. Mike is fighting like hell… although for Mike in his laid-back all-purpose shoes … he could kick it up a notch. His night last night … as I am learning was eventful…my friends, you want the nurse to tell you it was uneventful. I leave you with what my nurse Marjory told me tonight … he is holding his own. They have him on his stomach (which he has responded well to). He is stable. Blood pressure was an issue today. Right now, it is under control. I have told Marjory to whisper in his ear every time she is with him. I told her about what not only our community, but people far and wide are doing and she will tell him. We have picture papers being delivered tomorrow that we made this afternoon, so the nurses can read mine and my kid's messages.

I have never been so scared… but feel so surrounded by God, but also by this community. I beg you to keep praying. Keep thinking, he is worthy of our thoughts. I am ending with a few quotes and just one picture I will share from me before time. but it is Mike and Jesus the man who gave his life for us who will help Mike find his way back to us.

Be still I am fighting your battles.

God

Steady as we go.

It is ok if you can't handle everything today.

Love Sarah

Quote:

Life is remarkably interesting… in the end, some of your greatest pains, become your greatest strengths. Drew Barrymore

Scripture: Deuteronomy 31:6 "Be strong and courageous, do not fear or be in dread of them. For it is the Lord your God who goes with you. He will not leave you or forsake you."

Reflection: "To hold one's own" -to retain a position of strength in a challenging situation." The good news is as followers of Jesus, we will never have to hold our own because He promises to lift us up and to keep us. He is our deliverer our saviour and redeemer, our bright light in the darkness.

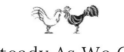

Steady As We Go.

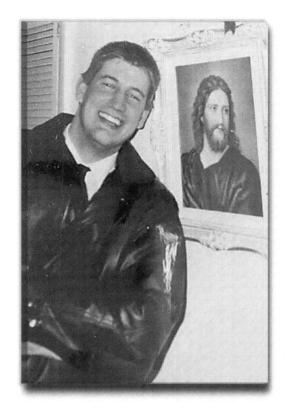

MIKE AND JESUS

"STEADY AS WE GO."

Day 8 /April 15th

I, and all our all-consuming thoughts are of Mike. To start I'm going to say. My husband, my kids' father is fighting for his life so if you are following me or do not believe COVID is real; if you are protesting anywhere about your rights to walk around town without a mask and how your rights have been invaded, if I hear of you I will unfriend you. Otherwise I ask you to unfriend me. I have no time for you, and you are neither Mike nor my friend. So, get rid of me now... or I will get rid of you.

To my true friends and to Mike's people. I saw Mike today (through proper public health and hospital procedures).

He is still our Mikey. I see him behind the tubes and the machines that are helping him to live. I'm not going to say what all I said to Mike. He knows the love. I told him to feel it. I will tell you the first thing I said that it is me, Mike. I'm right in the room with you. No phone laying against your ear. Not FaceTime. I am here.

I honestly don't think anyone has a concept of what these workers are doing. their tiredness, the doctors giving cell phone numbers. I am sure they never did before. But the love they have of their patients the comfort, the support system.

Steady As We Go.

Put this in your mind. I am garbed up as high as I can be to get to go in and see my husband, my soulmate my half. If you don't believe what I say is real leave my friends

I am tattooing on my body when Mike comes home 'Steady as We Go.'

Be still and let God.

If you aren't cheatin you aren't trying

If you don't think God has control over things ... look at what was over our farm tonight ... and although certain angels are with Mike, I have consent to tag Alida VanHamme. These people are doing a job you can't imagine ... will still try to tag.

Otherwise, God hears us... let him hear you!

Love, Sarah

Quote: When I felt myself slipping, you came with your love and kept me steady.

Scripture: Psalm 119:133 Keep steady my steps according to your promise

Reflection: Your faith in God is what will keep you steady on your walk-through life.

HOPE

Day 11/ April 18th

Eleven days now into this 'journey.' It is one I despise because I never wanted to be in this position or making these posts but now here I am... and I hope that you never have to. ... But this is about my Mikey/Mike/Chicken... and this is where day 11 took us today. Mike has continued with his baby steps. When I called for my before shift change call this morning nurse Lindsay told me that Mike was more aware, and they were balancing between sedation and pain. He had a good night. Mike also received a roommate yesterday. I know they must be a beautiful person in need of healing too.

Today was Nurse, Natalie. My first meet but once again...amazing. She reinstated that he was able to follow commands. Like squeeze my hand, wiggle your toes. He is triggering his own breaths using his own lungs more and the ECMO less... Amazing!

He has concerns and believe me... if I didn't have to post them I wouldn't but prayer for his white blood cell count to come down and blood in his urine to come down...... I don't want to post these private things about my husband, my best friend, my Mikey but I do KNOW that these steps he has had are because of the healing powers of God, faith, and prayer. So quite simply pray for lower white blood counts and that they may find out why there is blood in his catheter bag. He has the best of the best working on him.... He has a Covid team, a urologist team, an infection team... whatever team; they are there. They are incredible. I have never once left there without blowing kisses to these amazing people,

Steady As We Go.

crying, and saying that I know that Mike is in the best care he can be. I'm going to leave you with a story. I love seeing Mike. I need to see him. I do kind of the same things every time I see him. It involves tears, love, talking, reading Facebook posts, telling him how loved he is, how the farm, the barn, the fields, are all taken care of... I do not want him to have a stitch of worry, (it's hard to fill an hour conversation of one-sided talk). I talked about gas prices, how the wheat is greening up so nicely. Who all wants to have drinks... who wants to kick your ass for being here and hug you so deeply when you come home...Then I decided to sing (I told you he now has a roommate) so I sang, "The Gambler," with my heart (hoping his bed mate liked the song)? I sang as best I could. I finished that and told him how when I was in the driveshed this morning and first turned on the radio, "Sweet Caroline" was on, another favorite. So, I sang that one too. I think I was not too bad but when I turned behind, I realized that the door was open between Mike and his roommate and the room next with their 2 patients... and I think they eagerly anticipate my return tomorrow.

    Ok time to end but before I do - 2 things... Mike isn't done with us yet. Please keep praying. I know that God is hearing us, and I also believe that these amazing front line workers need a success story and I want Mike to be it. Please if you have faith, lift him in prayer. If you send positive thoughts, then please do. I could not watch but I heard our pastor described it as building a strong wall around Mike to protect. I know this is God. may he continue his miraculous healing. Finally Kaley E. Horton, and Kaley's Restaurant and "Kaley's Kakes". There isn't a more community, driven person. I thank her for what she has wanted to do...She is the meaning of small-town living, caring and passion. We are blessed.

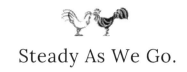

Steady As We Go.

Steady as We Go.

Baby Steps.

Gods Timing is Forever Accurate.

Believe it.

Trust it.

Allow.

Love, Sarah

Quote:

"*I learned that courage was not the absence of fear, but the triumph over it. The brave man is not he who does not feel afraid, but he who conquers that fear.*"

Nelson Mandela

Scripture: Isaiah 40:31 "But those who hope in the Lord will renew their strength. They will soar on wings like eagles, they will run and not grow weary, they will walk and not be faint."

Reflection:

Hope for Mike to continue to get well each passing day-for the need for the ECMO machine to end and for successful weaning.

Hope for his lungs to get stronger, and for him to be able to breathe soon without the use of a ventilator.

Hope for continued emotional strength for me, and our children.

Hope for recovery for Covid-19 patients in ICU's.

Hope for patients and families of Covid patients who are scared, that they seek refuge in you Lord and that you make yourself known to those who do not know you.

Hope for all of this and so much more.

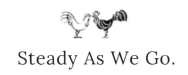

Steady As We Go.

BATTLE

Day 12/ April 19th

 Today life is trying to start back to school 'normal.' School is back in virtually and I am happy for the distraction for my kids. (Zack is working this year so he is waiting on time to get back to that). They need a little bit of normal to get by and to see friends online and to use their minds. I have talked about MY feelings and MY fear, but my kids are also feeling this fear. It is a tough time for all teens in this world... they aren't experiencing any of the joy we did as being young. It is saddening and it is heartbreaking to see them suffering because they know their dad is sick. Each of them, are being rock stars in their own way. but they are still kids who should be loving life, friends, and experiences.

 We are ending day 12... longest days of my life but at the same time. Time marches on. This is what I learned and say of Mike's day. Natalie was once again his day nurse. When I called this morning, she said that Mike is working hard (I know I say this a lot, but he is trying, and his body is fighting) and it is a battle of balancing his sedation with his pain. When he is more awake, he is more restless which affects his oxygen which isn't great for him with his lungs working so hard ...so today they sedated him more so that he can rest.... he does need a lot of rest. When I visited, I learned that they did another bronchi test and removed more fluid from his lungs. His antibiotics are helping his white blood cell count and the new catheter has greatly reduced the blood in his urine. I had another nice visit. Natalie is so caring. She takes the time to explain everything... even though I am sure she reassured me about the same thing yesterday. They have the time for you...more importantly, they have lots of time for Mike. I told Mike many things... to be honest I am sure I am repeating, but if I keep talking about love, fighting, prayer, friends, and family. I don't think it matters. I always pray for Mike, for his strength, for him to feel God's presence and for him to feel the power of prayer. I pray for the person answering the hospital door, to the laundry department to those amazing people working on his floor. I thought my audience might prefer the real version of "The Gambler," tonight, so I called it up on my phone and played it for him and our friends. I think they liked it too. To think that not only my Mikey, but all these people are battling for their lives... it is the quietest floor you could imagine. They wanted to prone Mike for the night (flip to tummy), so I told him I loved him our kids love him, as do all his friends... those who know and the many that have joined us on his journey of healing. I once again blew kisses to all these workers on my way out thanking them for everything they are doing for my Mike and everyone else, with tears running.

Finally at 6 my call to Natalie. Mike did well on the flip. He likes the time on his tummy. They will keep him sedated for the night. His oxygen levels are decent. So, I trust that until 5 in the morning when I call to see how his night was, I bow my head and pray that God will keep Mike safe until the next day. He is fighting so hard, I know ... keep going with baby steps. Individual prayers would be for continued lung improvement (obviously I guess but needed), white blood cells, still some blood in urine but also when he is less

Steady As We Go.

sedated... that he is not afraid... pray for calm and ease and peace so he can keep his oxygen levels where they were, and he can keep everything that is in his body still there. Natalie told me tonight he just needs some more rest... I believe her. But may we pray he be ready when they try again.

Two quotes from two wise friends tonight,

'There is always a door to push that can be open if you are strong enough to push it.'

'Patience may be the hardest of all virtues.'

Baby steps.

If you ain't cheatin you ain't tryin.

Steady as we go.

Love, Sarah

Quote: *"You never know how strong you are until being strong is your only choice."* Bob Marley

Scripture:

Deuteronomy 3:22

"Do not be afraid; the Lord your God himself will fight for you."

Reflection:

Let God fight your battles. He is your strength and support. He says to stand still. He's got it. Arm yourself with prayer and step out with faith. You are not alone. God is bigger and greater than anything you will face in this world. He will fight for you.

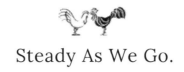

Steady As We Go.

WAIT

Day 13 / April 20th

Day thirteen is our day of rest. They continued to rest Mike this day so that when they feel he is ready again, his lungs will prove well. Mike proned well last night and then this morning they flipped him back to his back… (for those who possibly wonder how easy this could be, it takes about 6 nurses a half-hour all working together to achieve this procedure safely.) A simple move of a roll to a back to a stomach becomes a medical word called a prone.

Today's day nurse is Sarah. What a beautiful name! They turned him back to his back and he tolerated it well. Still, quite a bit of sedation, but they wanted him to rest. I visited with Mike today at 2. I met with a DR. from his team first and went over some questions and answers…. they are such smart and knowledgeable people! I then went to see Mike. Still my Mikey, just a more resting version… and I am fine with the rest, the doctors all say he needs it. Patience is the hardest virtue. My regular today… always how much, we and everyone else love him, a few things people asked me to tell him, about our kids, his brother, Cindy, and fam. His dad… I know they miss him. They talked about the possible snow, OHL season finally cancelled which gives him lots of time to get home for Ryan and Flint next year. Our kids are his dream. He loves each of them passionately, but this was his dream … and Ryan's and he needs to be here for that. Zack starting University, Holly starting high school with a strong hockey career ahead, Alexis also with gr 12 and hockey chances before her... This is what you live for! I prayed (always pray), sang for the gang and tapped his hand for all our love.

To finish I want to say that I have never seen workers like this before. They are overworked, they have never seen the volumes in the hospital like this in their careers, they are tired. I dare say they are scared but .... I have never seen a bicker or fight amongst colleagues, I have never seen anything other than professional respect, I have never seen anything but love and compassion for patients and families. These doctors and nurses I can see firsthand are fighting the fight of their lives. I ask everyone to be safe...because if these people get sick, who is our last line? We have no line. Think about that. We are down to our last line of defence. If you have a chance of a vaccine, take it. Help restore the world. I do not want anyone to ever be in the position I am in. 13 days of not hearing a hello, squeezing a hand, a smile, smart-ass comment, nothing but watching him lie still.

Small steps in the right direction can turn out to be the biggest step of our life.

1 Peter 5:10 - God always gives you all the grace you need. So, you will only have to suffer for a little while. Then God himself will build you up again. He will make you Strong and steady.

Baby steps.

If you ain't cheatin you ain't tryin!

Steady as we go.

Love, Sarah

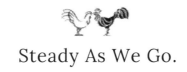

Steady As We Go.

Quote:

'Our willingness to wait reveals the value we place on what we are waiting for. Charles Stanley'

Scripture:

Psalm 130:5 "I wait for the Lord, my soul waits, and in his word I hope."

Reflection:

"When God says wait, he does not tell us for how long. When God says wait, we face one of God's greatest tests. When God says wait, we have decisions to make. When God says wait. We can only control two things; how we wait and who we become along the way." Waiting, waiting, waiting. God does not hurry things up-all in HIS timing. His promises are always fulfilled at the proper time. God transforms during waiting periods.

GOD PROVIDES

Day 14/ April 21st

Tomorrow will be 2 weeks since I took Mike to NGH. It is like a nightmare that will not end. For those who are sad and staying home, if you have a partner to do it with then do not be sad because you probably (I hope) have the most important person in your life by your side... so forget what is going on in the world, who you miss, who you wish you could see... and if you can see and talk to the most important person in your life. then be happy!

Mikey's day today. He had a mostly uneventful day (which is good). Rest as much as you can. Let your body be quiet and still. When I arrived at 2 for my visit x-ray was with Mike... they apologized for several times that I couldn't see him yet... you are helping Mike... you take as long as you like. I got in an hour after my time. I did not care. I only want to see Mike and to know he knows I am there... It is truly a small world... I know through friends a respiratory therapist who is on Mike's floor. I got to meet her, and she has her eyes on Mikey.

I just feel like I could talk about him forever so just know this. I love him. I love him in a way that stops me in my steps stops my heart, makes my heartache...but I BELIEVE.

My posts are long, I get thinking and talking. Prayers for specifics are that Mike, needs to be kept safe from secondary infections and to allow his lungs to heal.

Steady As We Go.

I also want to share the analogy a doctor today gave me... if you broke your leg the crutches the doctor gave you don't heal you. They are there to support you. So, think of Mike, these medicines are there to support him. They are supporting him until his lungs are ready, as do the crutches support the bone till it heals. (Wow these people just... I have no words).

Ok time to wrap it up. I want to be totally clear; I have a family, I have money. I have never been concerned about that. What is my concern? The most loving kind, you all know him. There are no words needed. So here is it...people feel better by helping, as we all do. I know how I am feeling day by day, sometimes second by second.

These fundraisers aren't about me. My family and I will be ok. These are about spreading the story of Mike. More people will pray for him, it will keep him a priority, more in the top of thoughts. I am so grateful for living in my small town. My life is about Mike.

These hospitals are so worthy. When Mike is home, we will decide what causes to donate to.

People want to feel needed; we all do. I guess I just need to say rest assured. I am ok but know that whatever money received will be distributed to a charity or whatever cause Mike and I feel fit. I get it. He is contagious, real vibrant, I can hear him talking in my ear. I just want him home. Keep loving him and thinking of him.

Prayer. Is the most powerful weapon against trials. The most effective medicine against sickness and the most valuable gift to someone else.

"It doesn't matter how slowly you go. so long as you do not stop."

"God gives his hardest battles to his toughest soldiers."

"Faith is taking the first step even when you don't know the whole staircase."

Steady as we go.

Baby steps Mikey.

Love, Sarah

Quote: *"Where God guides, He provides."* Isaiah, 58:11

Scripture: "And my God will supply every need of yours according to his riches in glory in Christ Jesus."

Reflection:

God always provides. He provided Mike with another hospital with an ECMO machine, kind and informative nurses, Fan 590 radio, a chaplain to pray for him as she walks by his room. God knows Mike's needs and he loves him unconditionally. God too knows your needs and will provide for your every need. God Provides-Tamela Mann "God Provides. He'll come through. When the clouds of doubt rain down on you, and test everything you thought you knew. Now you finally see what God can do for you."

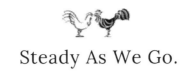
Steady As We Go.

BELIEVE

Day 15 / April 22nd

Many of my and Mike's group of friends are now being vaccinated. and I thank you so much. As I was talking to one of Mike's nurses yesterday, she said that the medical professionals and she herself are just saying get whatever vaccine you can. The risk of being vaccinated is far less than the consequences they are fighting right now.

They can treat the very few reactions to the vaccines. They cannot treat the multitude of Covid patients coming in. They are seeing the worst of the worst. I struggle to use the word 'lucky' currently with Mike... although those who know him know how lucky he is with his Superbowl pools or even his Roll Up the Rim his Tim Hortons streak. Is there anyone who loves sports more? But I do thank God that Mike got into the hospital when they have had a chance to learn, and before they have patients lined in the hallway.

This is what this day has taught me. Mikey's x-rays today show nothing worse. He was moving his arm and head a bit, but I didn't see as much agitation. Today while there I watched his nurses. Caroline today (lovely and beautiful). I watched them work on Mike, changing IV's, changing pads that are holding down his breathing tube. They are so caring and use such gentle hands when they touch him. These men and women care, take care of people with a kindness we don't fathom. I think... I know, that to stand in those hallway for 5 minutes would change your life. They wipe down his face with constant talk and chatter. I have told them all to call him Chicken. He may respond better to that than Mike! I saw them checking his ECMO machine to be sure it is doing its job... this machine is 1 man's job only and he is brilliant.

Mike has a roommate who was lucky enough to be unvented yesterday... So, I got to witness the next step... the physio. A whole new department but one I can't wait to meet! They too are compassionate and loving and caring.

I did my regular visit with Mikey. I read him texts, I updated him on sports, talked about our kids, told him his friend Pete Wybenga who also had covid (Pete came off vent the day before Mike went on). I don't think coincidence so his friend could have it. (He came home today... yeah Pete).

I told him how special he is. How I believe he is the only person I know who has that kind of reach... people are praying who never have before... being vaccinated who would have said no. Mike, My Mikey your Chicken ... He is reaching people, so I beg you to keep praying. Keep him at the top of your minds. He is not done in his earthly life yet.

Tonight, our eldest, Zack applied for a university residence at Brock. We did it, got through it (with help). These are memories, I need Mike to be a part of. For those who know Mike... and for those that are our new friends, I talked to nurse Caroline about how I know this is a marathon and not a race. I said that's ok, Mike has always hated running, he doesn't even really like walking and he would prefer to be with the pit crew at the end of whatever with a

Steady As We Go.

beer. That's our Mikey. A couple more things to share... some know I have been singing... singing and praying. Mike's roommate thank the Lord has been unvented so a lot more aware, but I cannot let that deter me. I hope she enjoyed the concert. I sang, "Hooked on a Feeling", "Oh Jean" and I ended with, "The Gambler", "The Gambler", chokes me up.

Finally, as I was gowning up to go in Mike's room, a male nurse respiratory therapist, whatever he may be came up to me and said... I was in the morning nurses huddle yesterday, someone read your post to us... thank you!

People give these people your ultimate credit your love your devotion. Mike's day nurse today is going home now to her 4 children aged 9- to 2-2-year-old twins. Pray for our world, pray for normalcy soon, get a needle.!

Specific prayers are that Mike's blood pressure be controlled.

His lungs can heal.

May we keep secondary infections away?

Calm and no fighting as sedation eases

...Mike's needs now include that the healthcare workers stay safe to keep caring... bluntly honest.

Quotes:

'When you need to believe nothing is impossible for your God 'and...

Joseph waited 13 years.

Abraham waited 25 years.

Moses waited 40 years.

Jesus waited 30 years.

If God is making you wait, you are in good company.

#Lightsonformike

Steady as we go.

Let go and let God.

Baby steps Mike.

Love, Sarah

Quote: *"When you need to believe. Believe, that nothing is Impossible for God." Unknown*

Scripture:

Mark 5:36 "Don't be afraid. Just believe."

Reflection: The definition of believe, "To feel sure of the truth." Believe that God is in control. Believe that the medicines and rest are healing Mike's lungs. Believe that his body will fight off anything else. Believe that something good must come out of an unbelievable time.

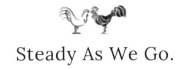

Steady As We Go.

COURAGE

Day 16 Friday April 23

 To be honest I am quite overwhelmed. I never thought when I made my first post scared for my husband's life, angry, terrified of this virus and so uncertain of my future.... I thought he would be home in a few days. Here I am 16 days later and now I have so many people following Mike's 'Journey'... I could never have even imagined. For those who know Mike personally, you know that he is the strongest person most of us know... so I decided if I expect him to fight this battle every day then I had best be prepared to pull myself out of bed in the morning and fight for him as well. If I am asking him every day to keep fighting, then there can't be any give up in me. He needs my thoughts and prayers. Along with everyone thought's and prayers. I believe they are going to be his saving grace. As many of you know I did a phone interview with CBC Hamilton today... they reached out to me and wondered if I would be willing to talk to them. How could I not do anything that spreads the word and the prayers for Mike and the awareness of Covid and these amazing health care workers. Samantha was easy to talk to and she pulled together the best features of Mike... the reasons we all love him... the reasons I am doing this.

 I also received a text from a special friend whose husband (and herself) mean a great deal to Mike. She and her work had designed t-shirts... steady as we go in honour of Mike...

I have Kaley E. Horton, with Chicken for Chicken... not only allowing people to share their love of Mike but less fortunate families have had dinners bought for them, community has been united. You can see the love... I think only Mike has the reach to accomplish these things. So, to say that my heart is touched by everything that is happening around my family, there are no words.

This is what I learned today. When I called for my 5:30 am call, I learned Mikey had an uneventful night... at that time it is really all I need to hear. Caroline was his day nurse again today. I spoke to her at 10 to see the plan for the day and to see when I could visit. 3:30 was good today. They were supposed to do a bronchi test on Mike, early in the afternoon and an ultrasound on his kidneys but when I got there the bronchi test had not been done yet... these doctors have so many things on the go, it had to be pushed till later most likely around 4:30. It was a busy day on the floor. Just action everywhere gowning up to get into rooms to check patients, monitor checking, double-checking, I can't tell you how much this crew works as a team. Doesn't even appear to be a captain... they all work as a crew. No one can have an ego here.

I was lucky enough to speak with Mike's doctor who will be with him for the next few days. He realizes how important and loved he is by everyone, and he ensured me that everything possible is being done for Mike... He spoke in the calmest voice, reassuring ... he said they continue to try to be proactive to find out what could go wrong before it does...reassured again. I now gown up on my own as sadly I know what I am doing and head in to see my Mikey, Mike your Chicken.

Steady As We Go.

Today he was resting but I still know he hears me. They had him more sedated for his bronchi. Mike still looks like our Mike. I tell him how beautiful he is and how I would love to crawl in that bed and lay with him. I read him some texts, I played him videos the kids made for him... I told him what a media sensation he is now (he would hate that!) I keep telling him about my Facebook because I know he hates it but secretly checks mine to see what is going on. I told him how much of a giver he is and how now he only needs to be a receiver... to receive all these prayers, energy, community support. You can be mad at us when you get home... for now, be a receiver. I prayed for him, his teams, for peace and calm for all people struggling and for healing to bring him home to us. I do laugh with him; I cry with him so my face shield is so fogged up I can't see anything. Just know he knows he is loved, and he is fighting, and he is going to win. I have no doubt.

A couple more things because people know I sing to him so some of the team starts bringing in the equipment to now do his bronchi tests. I say just let me know when you want me to leave, soon they asked me to go (so kindly).

I said, this is going to sound so stupid, but I always sing to him... can I sing 1 song before I go. They said of course. They were all gowned up and sterile so of course not going to leave so... for Mike and his six-person team who were in for his test. I sang "The Gambler." I gave him his love taps from our kids, all our friends, and me and carefully took my things off while I watched this team so carefully take care of my most important person.

I called when I got home to know that Mike's bronchi went well... they did not see any new issues in his lungs and not too much to cleanout. Here is praying for an uneventful night.

Individual prayer. Is to keep secondary infection far away from Mike.

Pray for his blood pressure and oxygen levels which are affected by treatments. Pray for his lungs and healing, pray for calmness, no fear, and a sense of peace.

Quotes:

Faith is like Wi-Fi. it is invisible but has the power to connect you to what you need.

When a train goes through a tunnel and it gets dark, you do not throw away the ticket and jump off. You sit still and trust the engineer. Trust God today no matter how dark your situation. God says, "You are coming out!"

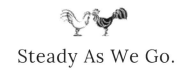

Steady As We Go.

As always:

Let Go and Let God.

Baby steps Mikey.

Steady as we go.

Love, Sarah

Quote: *What you are looking for is not out there. It is in you.*

Scripture: "Be strong and courageous. Do not be afraid. Do not be discouraged for the Lord your God will be with you wherever you go." Joshua 1: 8-9

Reflection:

COURAGE. The definition- "possessing or characterized by the quality of mind or spirit that enables a person to face difficulty, danger, pain." "From the doctors to the nurses, to the paramedics, to the respiratory therapists, the chaplain, the cafeteria workers, the cleaners, administrative assistants. You name it. COURAGE. These are frontline workers... people, who all day are caring for the sickest of the sick in a worldwide pandemic and then need to have a reserve of energy and care to bring home to their own families. The stress, fatigue, and emotional turmoil that they carry. The ones who leave the hospital and go cry in their car in the parking lots, the ones who use their own phones to enable families to see their loved ones-the ones who give a warm smile to visitors and the ones who take time to go above and beyond to care for their patients. They define courage. God- please continue to "EN-**COURAGE**" those who need courage. Lift them up in your name. Amen

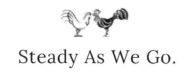

Steady As We Go.

BREATHE

Day 17 / April 24th

T his has taken a jump to a whole new level. I never thought that I would be an advocate for Mike... and what is now best for Mike and extremely important to me which is prayer, healing, vaccine awareness, covid reality and an awareness of our amazing first line/last line workers.

I learned last night that the article that I did for Samantha at the CBC Hamilton was among the most-read stories on CBC across the country. No surprise- Sam is an amazing writer and Mike is a newsworthy story. Here is the thing. Mike would hate every single bit of publicity that is coming his way. It is not his way. Don't get me wrong, he loves to be the spotlight of attention, for a quick come back, his quick wit that has you shaking your head, for a teaching opportunity in coaching, for a meaningful conversation that is making someone feel better, for a karaoke challenge. But never for something that he needs.

But now my focus is on what Mike needs. He needs to be thought of, he needs the hundreds of prayer chains that have started, he needs to hear the success stories that I read to him, he needs to be encouraged through thought and prayer.

I'm going to say, I told Mike today that there is one thing that he would think is good out of all this attention...

and that is, although Kenny Rogers, has passed on, my post regarding Mike's love of Kenny and "The Gambler" made Kenny's Facebook page. I'm sure Mike is thinking ... "Finally!"

When I first started Facebook I had two rules, I would only be friends with who I knew and I would not be 'kids' friends as I wanted to keep my adult life separate... well that kind of went out the window in the last few days... so I ask if you are now following me, that your interest is truly my Mike and his healing to recovery journey as well as my belief in vaccines, faith, and prayer and the health care workers. That is where it began, and where it continues.

Here is what I learned on this day. Mike had an uneventful night (yeah). The first night in many he wasn't proned and his numbers stayed consistent. Mike's day nurse again is Dianne. She has cared for him before but my first time meeting her. I was also able to meet again with his Dr. His ECMO machine is continuing the same level. His blood pressure was a bit more under control. They have him on some antibiotics to compensate for a need for additional platelets. All proactive in trying to fight any infection.

Again, today he was sedated. They do not want him too agitated because of the ECMO machine, and I trust everything they say. I have the greatest of confidence in these people's abilities. They know this is not a quick process, but they believe in Mike and their own abilities... (They are also all learning that he most likely responds better to the name, "Chicken" than Mike).

I had a nice visit with my Mikey, Mike, your Chicken today. He had his hair all cleaned up. He looked as he always looks, like Mikey. He was calm. I could see his chest moving.

Steady As We Go.

He is working his lungs a bit on his own. I told him he is social media famous. (Oh, he would hate this!)

I am going to say that today was my tough love day. I told him quitting was not an option. Nobody is quitting on him or doubting him. There is no other way than to listen to my voice and the thoughts and prayers of his friends and to start again with the baby steps home to us. (For those who know us... I am tough love) shake it off, and Mike is wrapping you in a hug and don't hold a grudging love. I told him we love him fiercely ... to receive our love and our prayers... the power of prayer. I so believe!! For this while you cannot be a giver Mike but a receiver. Let us all give back to you that you have given to us.

I prayed for him. For his recovering health, for the ultimate healer God to heal him back to his earthly home, with us! For peace and calmness and for his doctors and nurses and their families too. I read him some texts from friends, showed some videos and I sang for my gang. Today I sang, "Don't Stop Believing" (because I never will), "Oh Jean" because its growing on me and I now change the verse to I love him, "I love him, I love him," (instead of I love her). Finally, "The Gambler."

I heard this saying today. The way I see it ...yeah, I would survive it, but I might carry it to someone who wouldn't... and that folks is the problem. #Itsnotallaboutyou. My Mikey could be anyone (don't stand in this story). Please be vaccinated and be careful. Let's have a real-world back.

I gave him his love taps on his hand for his kids, his friends… those who he knew he had and the 700 he didn't (the price of people caring my Mikey) and for me who desperately is lonely, wants to hear your voice and hold your hand. I will see you tomorrow.

Specific prayers.

Please pray for blood pressure to be controlled and that Mike's lungs may heal. And that secondary infection be kept far away and pray for his peace and calmness.

Quotes:

Worry is like a rocking chair; it keeps you busy but does not get you anywhere.

Good things come to those who believe, better things come to those who are patient, and the best things come to those who do not give up.

#Lightsonformike

If you ain't cheatin you ain't tryin.

Baby steps Mikey.

Steady as we go.

Love, Sarah

Scripture: "The very breath of God is in you." Job 33:4

Reflection: Breathe as Mike takes in air; he is breathing in the Holy Spirit-the breath of life that is given by God. As he expels it, although he cannot talk-you are the air he expels-you are spreading the word of God and the power of prayer to our community and beyond.

Steady As We Go.

GRACE

Day 18 / April 25th

I know this is a far earlier post than I normally would do, but truthfully, I am exhausted. I am tired of crying, I am tired of being afraid, I am tired of being lonely, I am tired of being anxious, and I am tired of missing the most important thing in my life... what I am not tired of is believing... in Mike, in the power of prayer and miracles and in the knowledge and brilliance of Mike's medical professionals.

The time I was up this morning I watched an early morning church service, and the message was on ... The problem of miracles... do they still happen today. My attention was drawn. It seemed so appropriate. What I took from it is Jesus is more than a doctor or a magician, but an actual miracle worker. Jesus is still doing miracles, people are praying who have never spoken to God before, people who were not going to get a vaccine are getting them because of Mike, people are understanding that the front-line workers are being tried to their means. This is Mike. (No doubt to those who know him). So, I have no doubt that God is not done with him here on Earth... do not despair God is here.

I am not going to go into as much detail as normal today. Mike is still very much fighting his battle... ever harder... never giving up. He is working his hardest.

This is what I want you to take away from today... I am going to use limited medical terms. Mike is no worse today than yesterday. His lungs show some improvement. The doctors, the nurses, the medical staff have not quit in them as does my Mikey. Our issue right now is that he is bleeding too much through his urine (although as far as can see all looks fine in there). We need to limit the transfusions he is receiving. He needs to stay on the ECMO machine for the time being, so we need to find a way to do that while trying to decrease the bleeding.

They have a plan. It will be a great plan, we just need Mike to be strong for the next little bit... so without getting into huge details, they will clean his ECMO machine and will start to try to thicken his blood to reduce his bleeding, while monitoring oxygen and clotting. They were perfect in saying right now we are not worried in numbers; we are facing a bump in the road.

I had my visit with my Mikey... I did my regular... he knows I love him with my heart and soul. He knows the kids are the light of his life, he knows he has friends and family waiting for him at home. I prayed for him ... several times, I sang for him because I know ... or think he loves it, I touched his hand. I told him I loved him... to fight like hell because now is not the time to be tired or laid back, kick it up a notch I know you can. I read the farmer's prayer tonight to him. He is a farmer, the strongest I know so- you fight. I told him I will see him tomorrow. Love taps from all. Now is the time when I cannot stress enough not only the medical professionalism of these people but their compassionate care. beyond Mike, to me. I won't retell but these are beyond the normal people, these are angels in scrubs... there are not words to describe their compassion in my time of loneliness.

For my good news. I spoke with Dianne at 6 and she said that my Mikey, Mike, your Chicken took the circuit

Steady As We Go.

change like a champ. They have topped up his hemoglobin (we want it high). We want him to be as oxygenated as possible. His blood should soon start thickening a bit. His color and his oxygen were good. Mike still needs to fight. Fight of his life. we have been given a 'bump', but I know he can beat this too. Dianne was super proud of how he handled his afternoon.

Specific prayers for today:

Pray for strength for Mike.

Pray for the bleeding to stop.

Pray for the blood to thicken yet still be controlled by the ECMO machine.

Pray for complete healing for Mike to return home to his family.

Pray for COVID to be beat.

Quotes:

"Throw your lifejacket on and get in there and hang on."

"God has perfect timing; never early, never late. It takes a little patience, and it takes a lot of faith but it's worth the wait."

"Being deeply loved gives you strength; loving deeply gives you courage."

Steady as we go.

Baby steps Mikey

You ain't cheatin' you ain't tryin.

Love, Sarah

Scripture:

Ephesians 2:8 For it is by Grace you have been saved.

Hebrews 4:16: Let us approach God's throne of grace with confidence. So that we may receive mercy and find grace to help us in our time of need.

Reflection: Grace is "the love and mercy given to us by God because God desires us to have it, not because of anything we have done to earn it." We are to come to God freely and persistently, without fear. Seek, God and you will be gifted, grace.

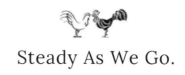

Steady As We Go.

FEAR

Day 19 / April 26th

    Today marks two weeks that Mike has been on the ECMO machine. Time does have its way of marching on, and I often wonder on which end it would seem longer... on the end of watching this or on the end of receiving this?

    I want to start by saying that I genuinely believe that every word I say to Mike, he hears. It is why they play radios or music to patients, it is why they take baby steps, it is why we are all still praying... because we believe in these patients' ability to hear us, whether through word or music and why we believe they have the power to feel the power of prayer around them.

    When I called this morning to Ann, I heard an uneventful night. Say no more. Yes, my Mikey you are doing what you need to do. Thank you for working so hard through the night, for enduring the changes you had to have made.

    Last night they moved Mike rooms. Not far, just two doors down but I can't imagine all the people required to get him to his new temporary home. The reason being that unfortunately there are 3 ECMO patients currently so they need for them all to be close so the ECMO man can diligently concentrate on all their machines. When I asked today what bed Mike is now in, they said 13.

For those who know Mike, what other number is he in than 13! His most favorite number, our kid's hockey, or ball number... as sad as it sounds, I was so happy! My special hometown nurse greeted me and led me to Mike's new room. I went in to visit. I am always awe-struck by how happy I am to see him again. How beautiful he is (I know it is going straight to his head), how happy I am to see him again. How relieved I am to see him again. He looks like Mike, only a quiet version. (This must be torturing him inside to listen). I miss his voice, a hand hold, a wink... but he is doing what we asked, he is fighting like hell. We knew we needed certain things over these hours, and he is doing his best... so here is what I know about my Mikey, your Mike, your Chicken. He is fighting. I see it in him.

He had an uneventful night. To be honest the plans for the next few days are to rest him. That's ok. He has only required 2 transfusions today compared to the 8 yesterday. His bleeding has slowed, his blood is thickening, and they are closely monitoring for clots. He is wearing special 'things' (my terminology not theirs) on his legs to reduce blood clot risks.

Nurse Sheila is amazing today... (what kindness and love she is reassuring and told me that today for what Mike is going through, what was expected of him, it is a good day! I spoke to night nurse Kale, as well. Steady as we go heading into the night.

Life is not easy right now... but it is not easy for many people... for where there is my story. And my Mike is another person's story. There are few beds left in this hospital, I won't say the number, but it is not reassuring. They are stretched to their max, so I thank God that Mike got in when he did.

Steady As We Go.

Ambulances keep coming in, choppers keep landing ... but the house is getting full... full.

For those who Mike has changed their mind on vaccinations, I thank you. For those that donate blood... I thank you. Mike has required 10 units in 36 hours, if you didn't donate what would we do? So, another request, vaccinate and donate blood. (I have always been accused of being bossy and controlling. I like things to happen like I say, so just do it!) I don't do that enough, but I will start... this too is saving his life.

Ok, ok I need to wrap it up. I am so happy that I got to see my Mikey again today. He knows he is needed; the prayers extend to 1000's. The nurses know he hates running and that he likes the beer at the end. This man will be their success story, He will be an answer to prayer, a nurse's struggle to care, this man will succeed. I ask of you to continue to hold Mike in your prayers, thoughts, prayer chains... he will be their miracle. He is our best friend.

Specific prayer requests for:

Healing of lungs.

Controlled bleeding.

Thickening of blood, but no clots.

A steady as we go, return to our life.

There is power in prayer.

"We could never learn to be brave and patient if there were only joy in the world."

"Even though I am in the storm the storm is not in me."

"If God put a Goliath in front of you, he must believe there is a David inside of you."

As always:

-steady as we go.

-baby steps Mikey

-get over the bump.

Love, Sarah

Quote: "My fear doesn't stand a chance when I stand in Your love"

Scripture: Psalm 56:3 "Whenever I am afraid, I will trust in you Lord."

Reflection: As you navigate through the storms in life, the "bumps" in the road, it is natural to feel doubt and fear. Remember you are not alone. God is your pilot; you are the co-pilot. Put your trust in him. He will lead you through the storm.

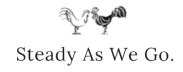

Steady As We Go.

GOOD FATHER

Day 20 / April 27th

Twenty days in. Spring is an important part of a farmer... as much as Mike has always worried how Kevin, himself and his dad would get all the farm work done, he truly always loves the tractor.

He is a farmer through and through. So, I am sad to think that he has missed the trees coming to bud, the tulips, the first grass cutting, even those stupid dandelions that we hate. I miss Mikey missing out on his favorite things.

We have had a decent ... not a good day. I refuse to get ahead of myself, but I want to give Mike the credit he deserves... he was put with some heavy tasks ahead of him. We knew the risks; I knew the expertise of his team. Some day distant in the future I will explain what Mike's body endured in the past 24 hours but know that. Wow...are these people smart.

My God in heaven they know what they are doing. They practice for procedures like this. The way my family practices hockey or fielding practices, these people practice their timing on saving lives. We have no idea their level of expertise. I will not talk right now in detail about them ... they have saved Mike countless times.

For today my Mikey, your Mike, your Chicken... he has impressed me all day, from my morning talk to nurse Kale and his calmness and yes it was an uneventful night, but he worked hard. To my morning talk with Natalie... yes, he is holding his own. They always have time for you, or you know when you can call back.

I visited Mike at 3 today... bed 13! I will be honest it's a bit of a routine now, I tell him how beautiful he is, how he is loved, I play him videos, I read the sports update, I tell him how much we have left to do here on earth. No one wants him in heaven yet. I tell him he can't be tired, to be a fighter... do you hear me? DO YOU HEAR ME??

I prayed for him, for the power of prayer for the friends he knew and the 1500 plus he has no idea. I prayed once again for the workers. I don't think anyone realizes their exhaustion, their tiredness, I don't know from their actions. I can see from their hallways.

One picture in your mind before I go. Mike is in ICU. Yes, he is critical care, but ICU is not Covid. They are running things a whole new way and I want you to picture this. Mike in his bed with his ECMO machine in his room. Everything else... all his machines' monitors, medications are in the hallway. they don't want to contaminate the room anymore than necessary. They monitor him from computers in the hall. Nurses communicate through thumbs up, thumbs down through the window to know what to do. They are nursing on a whole new level. they are learning and they are nailing it!

Let's wrap up... they thickened his blood enough to stop his bleeding for now.... yeah! His blood pressure is under control. Yeah. They are fighting secondary infections and they are confident in that. They are thinning blood again tonight for the ECMO machine to run to its best level and watching closely.

Steady As We Go.

Karen, Mike's nurse tonight is lovely... laughs, talks, they know he loves to be called Chicken.... Karen is updating him tonight on all sports, especially the Jays.

For my visit... some days are different, but I always tell him how beautiful he is, how many people love him beyond his wildest dreams, to accept the positive thought. I prayed for him and all. Told him we loved him... every single one of us. I gave him his love taps. For those who want to know the lineup today it was, "I'm on My Way," by the Proclaimers, then I sang "Lightning Crashes," because it is my favorite song and if I am going to sing your songs... then there must be something for me and truthfully, I can picture you belting this song out and it warms and aches my heart at the same time. I ended with "The Gambler."

I have one thing to say... I am accepting all Facebook, friends right now... because I want everyone to be thinking and praying of Mike. I have heard some awesome stories of which I will be sharing. Please don't 'wave' at me. Please don't send me a message saying, 'How you, doin?' You are not Joey Tribbiani.

That is not your place... It shows me that you are not my priority. I do this because I LOVE MIKE.

I am attaching some pictures tonight. the one picture of Mike's bed number 13... his most lucky number. Baby steps since being in this bed. The other is of the hallway outside his room for those questioning if they are busy. The halls are full of equipment and monitors, so yes, they are busy, to the max, pray for them. Be kind, wear a mask, covid is real, don't live my nightmare. The third is for hope. Steady as we go.

Specific prayer requests:

Continued lung healing.

Continued end to bleeding, please control secondary infections, and healing to come home, and to beat the bumps in the road.

Quotes: *"You gain strength, courage, and confidence by every experience in which you really stop to look fear in the face.*

"You must do the things which you think you can not do."

"It's hard to beat a person who never gives up."

"Practice the pause.

When in doubt pause

when angry pause

when tired pause when stressed pause?

and when you pause, PRAY."

"I may not be there yet, but I am closer than I was yesterday."

As always:

Steady as we go.

If you ain't cheatin you ain't tryin!

Baby steps, Mikey.

Beat the bumps.

Steady As We Go.

Love, Sarah

Scripture: Luke 15: 20-22, "You don't have to go to God with perfect prayers, the very moment you cry out, "Father," He runs to you and meets you at your point of need."

Reflection: "God is deeply in love with you and will never leave you. His love is relentless and healing. In our tumultuous and unpredictable world, we need to lift our hearts and worship our Good, Good, Father by reminding ourselves of who he is and what he does."

YOU NEVER LET GO

Day 21/ Wed. April 28th

Twenty-one days since this nightmare has started. Twenty-one days since I have heard your voice, or seen your eyes, or held your hand. Twenty-one days powering through the daily routine. Balancing between thinking about you, praying, putting negative thoughts away, and taking care of our kids. Our kids who are mostly the best parts of you. The fun parent as you always told me. I am always worried about grades and classes and following rules… you would always say go play hockey and do it better, not, did you do your homework, but did you practice your shot. I can't believe that you were ever the English award winner, but you made me believe it from day 1. I can't wait to see you now receive the French award as well.

I think maybe today I am just a bit sadder because Mike got a new roommate today. I don't know this man, I don't know how he lived his lifestyle, anything about his family, not even his name. What I do know is most likely 2 days ago he was talking and had lived in his body and today he lays there with all the machines and the quiet breathing of a ventilator.

He looks young, too young to be here, maybe 50. He looks to be handsome, but now here he is too… and it is heartbreaking. I can't even describe the ache that it is to see these patients. I do not know his story but neither Mike nor he, nor his two mates in the connecting room deserve the fight their bodies are enduring.

Steady As We Go.

I said to Mike. I think when you wake up, you and your roommate are going to be friends. I just feel you would like each other.

My Mikey, your Mike, your Chicken continues to hold his own. He is doing what he and they want him to do. He is resting. He is on very low blood pressure medications. They have thinned his blood again and he has continued to not bleed and little blood transfusions today. They will be trying to lower his heart rate so that his lungs can be improved. I asked Natalie who is amazing how do we get off ECMO... We need the lungs to do more of the work than the gas exchange on the machine. They will be slowly weaning it. Natalie is so patient with me and answering my questions, and with Mike. All in all, he is doing what he needs to do. They are not looking to wake him tonight, they need for him to be ready, so I believe he is readying for battle for the fight of his life. I have made it perfectly clear that quitting is not an option nor is tiredness. I have told him literally the thousands praying for him, feel the prayers... the love of family and friends at home... and not at home but everywhere, come home to your Simcoe home.

My visit is always the highlight of my day, and I am getting better at the one-sided conversation. I make notes on what to talk to Mike about. I secretly think he loves being "Twitter" famous. I talk about everything, but I will say as I looked at his roommate today. I had to wonder how did he and my Mikey get here? What the hell happened? How can these two strong men now be lying here silent? I think these two would be sitting sharing a beer in other circumstances...

(for those who know Mike we know he loves to have a beer with anyone and everyone... that's why everyone loves him) and I know someday these two bedmates will. Eye openers... yes, every day for 21 days now, but now I have two men relatively the same age battling their biggest battles. this is their Goliath; I know they each have a "David," inside.

Always the same, prayed with Mikey for himself, his healthcare workers, all the covid patients, for peace and earthly healing, family and friends, all patients on his floor. I talked, I sang... some new songs tonight. I am not sure who it was other than a farming lady who said someday you will be singing the Kenny Rogers, "Through the Years." I sang it tonight and boy oh boy the words. You were right. I also sang Tragically Hip, "Wheat Kings," with a smile on my face for seeing all our friends sitting around singing that together. I ended with "The Gambler" because I must.

One more thing before I go... as I was gowning up to go into see Mike, I saw the ECMO man (that's all I know him as, I do not know or do not remember his real name). To me he is the ECMO guy. I looked at him and said do you never get to go home? He says to me not very often. (He has the best accent, and he is just an amazing person, I love him for what he is doing). As I was leaving the ICU tonight, I passed him in the hallway, he had a tiny break, so I said, "Goodbye, thank you for everything you are doing." His response ... "No worries, you go home and get some rest." Oh my gosh!

I could ramble forever about Mike, his caregivers, their circumstances, the fact the covid unit is now full. But I will end with this. Enjoy your family and spouse, your best friend. Do not take a day or a moment for granted. I can't wait till Mike gets home; I am counting down the days.

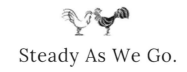

Steady As We Go.

Love, Sarah

Individual prayer requests:

Secondary infections be kept away.

May the bleeding be kept away.

For Mikes lungs to heal.

Let Mike's lungs do more of the work as they adjust the ECMO, machine.

For complete healing and return to us.

Quotes:

"Those who walk with God always reach their destination."

"Good things are coming down the road. Just don't stop walking."

"Winners never quit, and quitters never win."

As always:

Beat the bumps.

If you ain't cheatin you ain't trying!

Steady as we go.

Love, Sarah

Scripture "For God has said, "I will never fail you; I will never abandon you." Hebrews 13:5

Reflection:

God will never let go of you. You can be assured of this. He will comfort you and fill you with hope. He has a firm hold on you and will not give up on you.

When you think about God, it puts you in control, and is especially needed when the circumstances around you feel out of control.

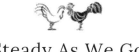

Steady As We Go.

"I NEED YOU"

Day 22 / April 29th

Every morning when I call the hospital to talk to Mike's nurse to see how his night was, I have been taking for granted that my report is uneventful... that is the only word I need to know. This morning I did not hear the words uneventful. I heard that Mike had a difficult night. They had trouble. Nurse Jessica who has been with Mike numerous times now was sorry to tell me that it was a difficult night. His oxygen was out of control. He was back on the rock; his blood pressure was not good. When I thought I couldn't find the new level of scared.... I found it this morning. I told Jessica that I know she did a fantastic job, I appreciated her, and I know she worked hard for Mike. I would call back later to see how he is doing.... I felt like I was on a cliff and didn't know whether to jump back or jump off. This has been one of the most difficult days of this journey. I received a call mid morn from Dr. Phillip, asking for my permission to do a CT scan on Mike's chest and abdomen...He does have some sort of infection, they need to sort this out. He wanted me to know the risks... but the benefits of this far outweigh any bad. I said to Dr. Phillip... You would not be doing this if you have given up hope on Mike so I know you are doing all you can... do whatever you need. Dr. Phillip responded, I have not given up on Mike at all, I am fighting tooth and nail and so is he.

Mike's nurse and I planned our visit for 4 today, enough time for him to go to his CT scan... this is a 7-man procession to get him to the scan and back. They clear the hallways of people so that they can get my Mike and all his equipment and his entourage safely there and back. It was walking on eggshells today. I spent a good deal of time on my knees in prayer.

But some good came of it... as much as I did not necessarily feel like it, I did the CTV Kitchener interview at Kaley's Restaurant. Mike deserves this additional support, as does Kaley E. Horton who my gosh... what a community supporter, what a ray of sunshine, what goodness coming pouring out of her heart. And the T-shirts... thank you Barb Harris and thank you The Custom Print Shop Company. It is so important to me that people understand what is happening and that is why I am doing these things. Because of my love for Mike and my belief in him.

So here is what I learned today about my Mikey, your Mike, your Chicken. I was so anxious going to see Mike today, so afraid of what I would find. When I got there, no fault of the hospital, I had to wait an extra 30 minutes which I went outside to walk then an extra 30 inside in which I got put in a private little room with walls to stare at. I am lucky that I have a cousin who works on Mike's floor, who came to sit with me... has been beside me this whole journey. So, this is what has happened. When I got in to see Mike, he has taken baby steps forward again. Thank you, God. His oxygen has improved on both ECMO and vent, his blood pressure medication is reduced again. He (and his team and God fought their way back!) He has not yet received his CT scan... sadly enough someone else was more in need of medical attention and Mike has been put on hold until tonight. But they took that time to change out some of his lines. He is reacting well to his antibiotics. I was just so happy to see him. While I got to see him, two nurses came in to take care of him

Steady As We Go.

and clean him... I only share this because I think it is so important for everyone to realize how far the care goes. Mike would not want anyone to be washing him (well in a normal life maybe he would.) These nurses cared for him and loved him and cleaned him and spoke to him. They apologized to me for taking my visiting time... I said never apologize for your care, you do what you are doing I am so happy I got to see this amazing side of your care. Love like he was their own. I'm not making this stuff up. I wouldn't want to, this is their lives, patient care is number one.

Today I basically told Mike I never want that phone call again in the morning. I told him again of love for him, the prayers he is receiving, the messages I am receiving, the vaccines being taken, the health care being appreciated, and ultimately the healing power of prayer to get Mike back to us. I prayed for him... harder than ever, I begged him to keep fighting, I spoke to it in my most stern voice. DO YOU HEAR ME! This is what I know. Mike would never quit on me. On us. I just need to remind him. Heaven does not need him. His mom would not want to see him nor would any other people he may know, they would want him to stay here with us and I keep telling him these things. He is soooo laid back in life. He can't be in this.

I felt good when I left. I was proud of him. I prayed, I sang, and I talked and don't worry, I told him the Leafs clinched their play-off spot. I want him on the parade route. This is their year!!

He is in the best hands. Doctors, God, and all our love and prayers. Mikey has this. Safe and well until another day.

Individual prayer requests:

Safe to and from CT scan tonight and for answers.

An uneventful night for Mike and his nurse, controlled oxygen levels, and blood pressure.

Prayers for his roomie and those in adjoining rooms, they all need it.

As always:

Beat the bumps.

Baby steps my Mikey.

Let go and let God.

Steady as we go.

Love, Sarah

Quote: "God is saying to you today. I know you are physically and emotionally drained. But you must keep on going. I'll see you through." Amen. "I need God in every moment of my life." "The struggle you're in today is developing the strength you need for tomorrow."

Scripture: Deuteronomy 4:29 "But from there you will search again for the Lord your God. And if you search for him with all your heart and soul, you will find him."

Steady As We Go.

Reflection: At the lowest points of our lives, God draws us into him. He makes himself known. Lord, we all need you-to smooth out the bumps in our roads. We need you in the good times and the bad. We need you all the time.

STRENGTH

Day 23 / April 30th

I am going, to be honest. I am not a blogger or a social media person or anything. I know nothing about this… So here is what I am going to say. I am mad right now because I had a post written, and I lost it. But that is not about Mike… so I will quickly re-write my day.

My Mikey is a trooper. He loves us all deeply. He has had some very rough spots these past few days, but I believe, and all of you must, he is taking baby steps back again. Mike had his CT scan this morning and they can see nothing of concern! Yeah, that is good news!! He endured the transfer there and back. I got to visit Mikey at 3 today. Leslie is his day nurse; I haven't met her until today. She is wonderful. They are weaning Mikey from sedation, so this is what I learned about my Mikey, your Chicken your Mike today. I learned he is a fighter, as we all knew. I learned he can fall behind and bounce right back. I learned that prayer is a big power, as is God, as is his medical team….

I got to witness an x-ray for Mike's roommate.

The expense and magnitude of this machine… is incredible, they said I could stay while preparing but then I stepped off to the side with the other two crew. Did you know the average age up there right now is 30-60…? 30????

How can anyone not believe this is real? How can people be protesting the most silent wing in the whole hospital with people working tirelessly to save lives? I can not even tolerate my anger. I must save my energy for Mike

Steady As We Go.

and the crew. Stupid can't be fixed and stupid will not stay 6 feet apart.

But now I am taking away from the best part of my day. Mikey moved his hand towards mine, he slightly opened an eye. I saw his eye for the first time in all these days. I always knew he heard me. I guess if anything because I know so many people are following me. Be proud of my Mikey. I love him with my body, my heart and soul but believe in the health care workers. My gosh. I saw some things today, they love, they talk, they teach, they care. The thing is someone is going to come in there who didn't believe in them. Will that be your person, your lover, best friend., husband, father? I pray to God this is not your story.

Prayers for tonight:

Secondary infection can be controlled,

healing of lungs.

Earthly healing for my Mikey.

Quotes:

"If You're praying about it,

God is working on it."

"It's hard to be a person who never gives up."

"You're only as strong as the table you dance on, the drinks you mix, and the friends you roll with."

And as always:

Steady as we go.

Beat the bumps.

If you ain't cheatin you ain't trying

Baby steps my Mikey.

Love, Sarah

Scripture: Philippians 4:13 "I can do all things through him who gives me strength."

Reflection: Are you tired? Worried? Anxious? Is your strength depleted? God can help. Pray. God will answer you and encourage you.

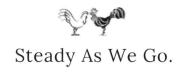

Steady As We Go.

HALLELUJAH

Day 24 / May 1st

A new month today, a turn of the calendar. Who would have thought that life could still pedal on? But it does and in my eyes, Mike is 25 days closer to being home. Tara was Mike's night nurse both last night and tonight. I have never seen her, but her voice is so upbeat and confident. Mike had an uneventful night last night. Thank you! Go home and get some sleep.

I couldn't talk to his day nurse due to rounds until 11. So many things flash through your mind while you are waiting. When I finally had a chance, the Charge Nurse answered, I said who I was and that I just wanted to see how Mike's day had started, and she told me that Karen, was his day nurse, she was in the room with Mike, his eyes were a bit open, and she would rather sit with him and talk than come to talk to me... yes you have your priorities straight Karen. You are where you should be. The Charge Nurse confirmed that 3 would be a good time to visit.

Today I spoke to the Haldimand Press (my good old hometown paper). I just feel it is so important that people be aware, and I want everyone to know about Mike. He deserves this time. I appreciate the people who did not know him wanting to know who he is.

This is what I learned today about my Mikey, your Mike, your Chicken. Mike has had a steady as you go day. He has taken no steps backwards. He is working hard... I can see it in his chest. The challenge to breathe on his own. Not the steady rise and fall that we all enjoy watching and feeling but a true work at it. I told him first how beautiful he is. Secondly how proud we all are of him. Many people have joined this journey and although I know you do not know Mike or I personally, I know you have a vested interest through prayer in his recovery. Some have asked to meet Mike after. (I told him he is going to be busy).

It is busy up here today.... it's not like, a Tim Hortons long line up or waiting for a cashier in the grocery store (don't misunderstand these are important jobs too), but it was action today. So much happening, so many unwell, so many such intelligent people knowing exactly how to treat these people.

I only know four who I call my crew, but every two rooms are full of a crew. They scurry, they garb up, they leave, they garb up 1 minute later to re-enter. The x-ray machine was back today for my crew in the adjoining room. Mike's roomie had an ultrasound. They do not stop, and they do not stress. I spoke last night about the age of these new covid patients, the average age is 40! 40 and on a vent fighting for your life.

I'm scared, the health care system is scared... because they are bursting... to be honest and I am not a swearer. This is a f#&kery! They don't stop. I know, I have no anti-covid followers, following me because I read every comment... I honestly do. You put the time into Mike. I want to see your positive energy, but I would challenge any anti-believer to confront me.

Steady As We Go.

My time with Mike... busy in the room as you know but I told him all the happenings. My brother and sis, Ange sent videos for him to hear, and my nieces Corah and Hannah sent videos. They are coming home at Christmas and Hannah has promised Uncle Chicken cans and cans of "Bud Light... she knows the way to his heart.

I think we all know the drill by now. I pray for everyone and everything but an extra measure for Mike. Told him stories, told him how his neighbor down the road is losing his mind and hurry home cause Ireland Road is going to hell! I sang, "Wheat Kings," "Can't Stop Believing," "Oh Jean," and "The Gambler". I am going to be so ready for the karaoke bars with my team this summer.

I tell him he is needed in his earthly home and his mom does not want to see him (as hard as this is, I think it is important). Told him of his strength, the love and prayers being poured out to him, and I told him I am a little bit famous. Sorry, but you made me be. Motivational speech always, don't be tired. You are not a quitter; you work my Mikey, and I WILL SEE YOU TOMORROW.

For those who know him. I know you love him; for those that didn't - I know you now love him.

To wrap-up my friends, keep the faith, keep the prayers. keep the love. I know Mike is coming back to me and we are all going to be better people because of what he has taught us. Thanks for joining me.

Individual prayer requests:

Pray for lung healing.

Pray for no more secondary infections and the controlling of them and the doctors and nurses continued proactive treatment.

Pray for Mike's calmness. For Mike to get off his vent, he is going to be uncomfortable for perhaps days. He needs to be calm. Pray for understanding for him, for the nurses to walk him through and that he feels our love, prayers, and peace. Also keep Uncle Chicken safe and well until another day.

Quotes:

"God is soooo much for powerful than Covid."

"Sometimes our lives have to be completely shaken up, changed, and rearranged to relocate us to the place we're meant to be."

"Give it to God and go to sleep."

As always:

Beat the bumps.

Baby steps Mikey

Let go and let God.

Steady as we go!

Love, Sarah

Scripture: Revelation 21:21, "Everyday we need to raise a Hallelujah to Jesus Christ, the One and Only God, the God who is One, the God who allowed himself to be crucified so that we may spend eternity with him on the street of gold."

Steady As We Go.

Reflection: Make worship your weapon to battle storms in life. The worship song "Raise a Hallelujah" was written for a 2-year-old boy, who was in ICU with an E-coli infection and not expected to make it through the night. Sometimes singing a little louder will help drown out the unbelief. Never give up in the middle of terrible trials as nothing is impossible with God.

COMFORT

Day25 / May 2nd

As I look at my wall tonight before I write my post, I am overwhelmed. I can look to it for love and support. I can look to it for prayers being written for Mike or my family. I can look to it for encouraging stories people are sharing with me... stories of miracles, stories of healing, stories of hope. I can look to it to see how Mike has impacted everyone along on this journey in some way and realize once again how lucky I am to call him mine.

It appears that Mike does not like Sundays... He had a rough day last Sunday and today was not his best day... Before I give you details, I want to be specifically clear that neither myself, my family, or Mike's doctors nor God have given up on Mike. Just the opposite... it is time to get specific! Everyone is still fighting tooth and nail; the lifejackets have been thrown on for Mike and the whole floor. We knew there would be ups and downs, which make us sad and deflated but this is not the time for that... so please don't let your minds wander in any direction. Stay focused on healing and recovery and ultimately for him to come home!! I am telling you all this because this is as it is... he will conquer but basically, every ounce of prayer is going to help Mike... that is why I share with you.

So, this is what I learned today about my Mikey, your Mike, your Chicken. Dani is Mike's Day-nurse today and she is kind and has a gentle voice. Mike has needed to be increased again on his oxygen. His X-rays of his lungs aren't showing a great deal of improvement, which they had hoped for more by now.... OK, I need to go in there and give my best

Steady As We Go.

speech I have ever done. I will tell him how important, how loved, how needed he is. I love this man... I will do anything for him. I will tell him his importance to everyone... I will tell him his kids need him... I will tell him I need him... I know he knows all this, but I will tell him again. My visit is always my day's highlight... to just see him, to touch his hand, to know in my heart that he knows I am there.

Mike's doctor came in while I was with Mike... God bless him I do not want to be in his position... having to talk to families about critically ill patients, having to answer these questions, having to move to the next bed and do the same thing again. I believe in Mike, the power of prayer, and in these doctors and nurses but more prayers...lots and lots of prayers would be great now. Mike has been on ECMO for a long time now... the longer he is on it, the more other issues we will face. Mike's lungs are still damaged... as his Dr described we need them to 'pop back' so that they can start to function better. Get better control of his oxygen. I know how wonderful this doctor is and I told him that I know he is working so hard, and he has my most important thing in my world in his care... I shed some tears... I shed a lot of tears every day and I told him I just don't understand how we got here... I don't understand how this is where we are right now. How is Mike the patient in this bed... how am I the wife standing here having these conversations. I told him I don't know how you are doing what you are doing... look around you, these are four young bodies lying here... this crew... how can you not be so sad every day. But he is. But his desire to heal is bigger. Today's post is difficult. Nobody in that hospital has given up on Mike... they never will. I won't, you won't but I told Mike it is time to start making some steps... the time to be laid back is over... time to jump into action... time to run on the diamond when you disagree with an umpire's call, time to get right up to the boards when you have 'an issue' with the ref. It's time to get off the left-field fence and get in the ball game.

We all know what I did today in my visit... I prayed... long and hard, I talked to Mike... he is just so damn beautiful to me. I touched his hand, I felt only one song was needed today and that was "The Gambler." I told him how much love and prayers are being thrown on him... heaven is being stormed!! I know it is. I love tapped him and I told him I would see him tomorrow... I will be back tomorrow.

I just want to say one thing... I believe that God is the ultimate healer and miracle worker. I believe he has given these physicians and nurses the greatest gift he could ever give to anyone. But I believe that in God all things are possible. God, I ask you, in the way that only You can do, to restore Mike's lungs... may they 'pop' as the doctor wants. May he stay safe on ECMO, and may you heal him so that he can be off it very soon. May you be with his oxygen. There is power in prayer God. I am asking you to start this miracle happening. Please bring Mike to earthly healing... his mom does not want him there... push him back dear God, make him a fighter for where you have put the Goliath of Covid in front of him, you have also put the David inside of him. God bless the power of the prayers... lay them on Mike, breathe into his lungs. Bring him back to his family and friends. I believe and I pray my most fervent prayer. I ask you all to do too.

Individual prayer requests.

Healing, healing, healing of Mike's lungs.

Steady As We Go.

ECMO machine, make him strong enough to come off.

Prayers for these amazing doctors and physicians... I cannot say enough about them.

Quotes.

"WHEN GOD STEPS IN MIRACLES HAPPEN."

Be still. The Lord will fight for you; you need only to be still.

Exodus 14:14 "And one must understand that braveness is not the absence of fear but rather the strength to keep on going forward despite the fear."

As always,

You got this Mikey.

Steady as we go.

Prayer is strong.

Love, Sarah

Scripture: 2 Corinthians 1:3

"Praise be to God, the Father of all compassion, the God of all comfort who comforts us in all our troubles."

Reflection: God blankets us with all the comfort we need with all the troubles we face.

JUST BE HELD

Day 26 / May 3

Over these last 26 days, so many people have reached out to me, I have heard stories about Mike that I did not know existed. I love hearing how much he means to people, what he has done for them, how he has changed them, made them laugh, made them feel better and happier and made them stay... for "Just one more" with him. I try to share memories with Mike... a lot of our best times are with family and friends but every memory of him makes me smile. I am confident we will have these memories again... but it is the memories of Mike with his little strut, his smile, his love of people, and being with everyone. It was always a joke that we could not tell Mike our cottage week in Turkey Point until the day before we were to go... because he would invite everyone for a drink on the deck... I would be cooking dinner for every Tom, Dick and Harry and Mike would be out on the deck laughing and just having a great time... I caught him one morning inviting the garbage man to the deck for a drink after he was done work... really my Mikey. He has always been like that, giving, generous with everything and I just can't wait for us all to take care of him when he gets home... because I believe he is going to be doing just that.

So, this is what I learned about my Mikey, your Mike, your Chicken today. Mike had an uneventful night with nurse Stephanie. She told me about Mike but then also asked about myself and the kids. She is amazing. Day shift today again was Dani. Once again, a busy day up there. There has been not much change since yesterday. He is sedated. He did have a bronch today and he did tolerate that. His roommate while

Steady As We Go.

I was there today, was getting moved to another hospital... I don't know why but I got to watch the preparation of getting him ready to go... the care and thought it takes into packing wires up, the ECMO machine, the oxygen... the moving of this man from bed to stretcher. Nothing is easy up here. There are only 8 ECMO's available currently at Mike's hospital and 7 are being used. Can I also tell you that they are preparing for waves 5 and 6... and yes, we are currently only on wave 3!

Procedures are being done on all these patients; they are going constantly. I wish you could all witness it... but then I really don't because this is not the place, that I would want anyone to ever be at. I talked to Mike; told him I love him. I concentrate so much on myself and my kids and how we are missing him... but I want you to know Mike has a dad who is struggling not having his morning talk with Mike. We lost Mike's mom Tina to her battle with cancer this past July. Mike, therefore, I say that your mom would not want you to join her yet... she never would, she was a selfless person. He has a brother and business partner who is missing his partner, not to mention a sister-in-law and three nephews and niece. He has my mom and dad who are living this nightmare and he has my brother and sister-in-law and two nieces on Vancouver Island feeling about as far away as they ever have. He has friends ... my gosh does Mike have friends, who I know are openly aching for the loss of not having him here right now. Why are we sad? Mike makes us all feel good and that is why we continue this because a guy who can make us all feel this way is going to pull through this and then say, he had it the whole time. I talked to Mike, I prayed for Mike, prayed for improvement, prayed for lung healing, miracles, for the feel of the power of prayer. I showed him some videos. I motivational spoke again… some might call it yelling, I call it motivational. Time to pick it up Mikey, more fight in you… never going to doubt you or give up. The room was a lot busier and loud today so I thought today I would play songs and sing with them, so I did "Oh Jean" and I did "The Gambler" for him tonight. I never want to leave him; I would stay forever but I told Mike I need to get home to the kids until he can get back to help me… because I know you want that as much as I do. I gave him his love taps and said I will see you tomorrow. You be good and baby steps my Mikey.

To be clear again tonight. I share this because Mike has prayer needs and healing needs… There is no give up on the steady as we go crew. God is in control and God has made some amazing … no wonderful, doctors and nurses that have blessed these halls. I see Mike working. I see them working, cleaning, loving, sanitizing, caretaking, doctoring… go home repeat. As I left Mike's room tonight his ECMO man was there (I do not know his name but I kind of like just calling him that) … he says to me… are you ok, how are you? The extended level of care, and I must say I got asked that 3 more times before I made it to the door… Mike is my fight, but these people are my care… My Mikey needs them, and I pray to God you never do.

Specific prayer requests:

Secondary infections please be kept at bay and controlled.

Complete healing of his lungs that they 'pop,' please pray for healing to return home to us.

Steady As We Go.

Quotes: *"The tiny seed knew that in order to grow it needed to be dropped in dirt, covered in darkness, and struggle to the light."*

"Every strike brings me closer to my next home run."

"You've got what it takes, but it will take everything you've got."

"Faith… it does not make things; it makes them possible."

As always:

Beat the bumps.

The Lord is on my side I will not fear.

Baby steps my Mikey.

Steady as we go.

Love, Sarah

Scripture: Isaiah 41:13, "I am holding you by your right hand-the Lord your God. And I say to you, "Do not be afraid, I am here to help you,"

Reflection: There are days, you just need to curl up into a ball and just be held.

… Author Sarah VanNetten

CORNERSTONE

Day 27/ May 4th

As sad as life is right now, as much as every day… most every moment is crippled with a fear I did not even know was possible, a fear of not knowing how I will get to the next moment. I worry for our kids and their feelings, there is good happening. We just must look a little harder. Two different articles about Mike were shared on Facebook today and I am so proud of them both. The Hamilton Spectator, when I did this interview on Sunday, I appreciated the ease with which J.P. asked his questions. He was sincere and openly interested in getting to know Mike and what kind of person he is. I expected just an article somewhere in the paper. I did not expect to see my beautiful Mikey's face smiling back at me from the front page. This picture captures his EVERYTHING! It shows his ease, his confidence, his love, his sparkle, his love of hometown wearing his folk sweatshirt and whenever possible a drink in his hand.

The Hamilton Health Sciences article is a whole new level. Its feature is the ECMO machine, and the brilliance of the machine is amazing. That they chose to use Mike to show how real people can find themselves in this situation was an honor. Here is the thing. I will talk to anyone to promote what I have come to believe in, the power of prayer, the reality of COVID, that I love Mike with my heart and soul and want more people thinking of him and praying, and finally these health care workers…the unstoppable beasts working to save our people.

Here is what I learned today about my Mikey, your Mike, your Chicken. Greg was his night nurse last night and

Steady As We Go.

when I spoke to Greg before 'bed' he said he had times of recovering his oxygen. They have put him on dialysis... they want to be sure to keep the fluids moving through Mike's body... again trying to eliminate any problem we may encounter. My morning call to Greg was "uneventful" ... perfect Greg, thank you for your care go home to sleep. My visit today was again at 3.

When I arrived on the floor to get gowned up, Chaplain Claire was at the nurse's desk. Claire considers the ICU her special home so can often be found wandering these halls. We spoke for a few minutes. I take comfort in her and in her opinions and thoughts and her clarifications. She told me that she knows many people who have used singing as a healing method with their loved ones. I said Claire I sing to him every day here, (let's get this straight... before all this, I was never singing to Mike every day, we occasionally did a karaoke duet, but this is a whole new thing for me). Claire said wonderful but know that apparently hymns and Christmas songs are great because they go to the comfort spot of a person are wonderful. Thank you, Claire, and please keep praying every time you pass bed 13.

Pam is Mike's nurse today. They did lower his sedation a bit this morning and he was able to follow their commands, he slightly opened his eye... yes, he is still fighting! They did up it again as they don't want to 'rock the boat' right now. They changed out a bunch of sites... must be so careful of infection. They had tried to clean Mike up a bit before I arrived, but he just wasn't in the mood for it at that time, so they didn't bother.

I had a good visit with Mike. I tell him all the reasons he must live (I know he is aware of them, but I must remind him) I told him that I'm sorry, he can be so mad at me later, but he is the Spectator, front-page story... and yes, I am sorry there is a medical article featuring your ECMO machine and you. He can hate me later. I played him some videos of friends talking to him. I prayed for him as always for earthly healing, for miracles for perseverance, for strength, for angels to fight to keep him here... there is no tiring Mikey. When you get tired, you think of me, and I will shoot you every ounce of energy I have. To be honest, I told him I hate those blessed chickens, I don't want to learn to drive a tractor... you come home and do these things... this farm was your dream, not mine.

Come back home to live your dream. To be honest I listened to Claire... I didn't think I was capable of hymns (emotionally) yet, and so many beautiful Christmas songs are so slow, so I sang (I think I may be on the crazy watch), but I sang "Rudolph the Red-Nosed Reindeer." What I won't do for you, my Mikey. I followed it with "Wheat Kings," and "I Can't Stop This Feeling." I did not have time for "The Gambler" as the next nurse came in to draw blood. I wish I caught her name but young again, the second day here, she has come from McMaster but because they are not doing pediatrics, she has been deployed to Hamilton General. She is so spunky. She told me she has been talking and singing as well to Mike all day... she sings along to the radio that plays in his room. We had a little conversation about Mike and to Mike. While she was still doing her work, it was time for me to go... I told Mike how much he is loved, he is needed, he is wanted. I gave him his love taps with all the love I must give. Their plan was to x-ray Mike and to get him cleaned up... so I told him he had better cooperate with them for a clean-up. I would very much

Steady As We Go.

like to see him looking a little fresher tomorrow, do not give these girls a hard time... the nurse's response was "Yes, Mike, happy wife, happy life!"

As I was de-gowning in the room she came over and had such an interest in the pictures of our kids on Mike's wall. They all want to know him as we do. I thanked her, told Mike I will see you tomorrow, and left.

One last thing to leave you with, as always someone always asks me how I am... tonight it was a nurse Mike had a few days ago. She told me to be sure I am taking care of myself because I have a long road ahead of me. I said that I know it is a long road and I am so ready for it... he is not giving up. She responded, "I believe you are right, and I believe in him... he has not stopped fighting yet, he will not give up. I believe he will beat this." Thank you! These workers believe, he is so strong. There were so many good success stories sent to me today. Heaven is once again being stormed. I will see you tomorrow my Mikey.

Individual prayer requests:

Full healing of his lungs. May they "pop."

Healing through God and these amazing workers.

Secondary infection be kept far, far away.

The power of prayer be heard.

Oxygen levels improving.

Tonight's quotes:

"Winners aren't people who never fail but people who never quit."

"Where there is great love, there is also miracles."

"Faith is to believe what you do not see; the reward of this faith is to see what you believe."

Get off your all-purpose shoes Mikey and get your runners on!

As always:

Beat the bumps.

You've got this, my Mikey.

Steady as we go.

Love, Sarah

Quote: "Christ alone, my cornerstone. Weak made strong, in the Savior's love."

Scripture: "Behold I lay in Zion a stone for a foundation, a tried stone, a precious cornerstone, a sure foundation."

Reflection: In every stone building, one stone is crucial. It is laid first and ensures that the building is stable. It is the rock upon which the weight of the entire structure rests-it is the cornerstone. Jesus is the "Chief cornerstone" of our faith. He is our rock. I pray today that you continue to stand firm on this rock; that Mike is made strong through his Saviour's love. If you stand with, Jesus, you stand on solid ground.

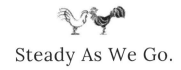

Steady As We Go.

WHILE I WAIT

Day 28 / Wednesday, May 5

Each morning when I get up, I think today is a new day... please let it be a good day. Please let this be a day of improvement. This is now a life where you hate the sound of your phone ringing, (I have people who know to text me before they call me. Then I am OK.) The sound of the phone sends panic running through me, my kids jump at the phone ringing. I would far rather call for nurses' updates than to have them or doctors call me. It's all the little things, the things you did not realize you would even miss until they were gone. I kid you not, I hate doing laundry because there are not any of Mike's clothes to fold, I am not picking up his barn clothes from the floor. Not moving his shoes from the middle of the front hallway or reminding him to take his lunch pail to work in the morning.

It means nothing, but every morning all Mike had to do to go to work at 5:30 in the morning, was take his cell phone and his lunch pail which I always got up and filled for him to leave the house. I can't tell you the number of times and he went out the front door, put his pail onto the rocking chair outside to shut the front door... and that's where it would stay. I would take a pic of it when I found it and send it to him and say... so close Mikey. I would text Mike to tell him he forgot his lunch, only to have his phone ding on the pillow on our bed. Then I would text his good friend, "Too Tall" at work and say tell your buddy his lunch and phone will be in his truck in half-hour. For those who know Mike... this is just him... laid back, no concerns, easy or should I say "Steady as he goes."

So, this is what I know about my Mikey, your Mike, your Chicken today. At 5:30 this morning Carla told me an uneventful night. Thank you, Carla.

Mike's day nurse today is Stephanie who we have had before. Stephanie called me this morning (heart sink and panic), but it was ok. Mike has had no change; she is calling me to tell me (as she knows I visit every day) that I cannot go in the room. Mike has a new roommate, but he is on an open oxygen system (meaning he is not vented but in caution, I cannot go in), so if I want to see Mike it will just be a view through the window. I told Stephanie I don't care if I just look at him for 15 minutes, I need to see him. Her response, see you at 3.

When I got to the hospital, I met with nurse Stephanie. I want to be clear, as much work as Mike has yet to do, we must celebrate his baby steps, because that is what we have prayed for and asked for, so we need to celebrate them and then move onto the next steps we need. So today, celebrate what I tell you... be proud, keep praying but acknowledge, yes Mikey, you did good! So today Mike did this... he was able this morning when his eyes opened to acknowledge Stephanie. She asked him if he understood her, and he gave a little nod. She told him she knows he is scared but to not be tired and keep fighting... He is FIGHTING!

When I arrived, I learn a few more steps. His oxygen on his vent is the lowest it has been. By making some other adjustments on his vent, they are forcing his lungs to 'pop.' They are adapting. I just want to say, I know I have a lot of medical people reading my posts right now and I know I am

Steady As We Go.

not describing it exactly how I should, I am trying my best but don't ever be afraid if I am saying something incorrect to help me in speaking it better. I have the good fortune to have a cousin and what I feel has now become a good hometown friend on Mike's floor. And they have been amazing... sitting with Mike, encouraging him... telling him to get his ass home. So fortunate to have this support.

    For today's visit I took Mike's phone with me and then I called his phone and had it on speaker and nurse Stephanie put it by his ear. I had just a half hour to talk to him as then the curtain blinds would be turned so procedures could be started on the crew. I thought I had experienced the utmost awkwardness within his room... talking to him, crying in front of people, singing to strangers... but, guess not. Now I am in the hall looking through a window, talking into my own phone, so all the hallway workers can hear, and the speaker phone on by his ear and man did it magnify! I could hear myself in the hallway. It gets to the point you don't care who hears what you are saying, you are only talking to one person, and you have a limited time to tell them everything that is important. So, I told him we loved him, I told him again all the reasons to live, saying again Mikey I know you know this but here is your reminder. I prayed for him, thanked God for the baby steps we have asked for. Prayed for everything and everyone, for ultimate earthly healing. For the doctors and nurses... for his roommates. I told him about his kids again and their doings and what we will watch them do, about his family, the chicken crop we just shipped. Told him about the "Jays" and about the "Astros" and the "Yankees" game last night. How so many people love him. I told him we are proud.

Fight like hell. If you are tired then reach to me, reach to us and we will give you every ounce of strength we have.

I told him I believe in miracles, God performs them, these doctors and nurses are the instruments, and we all need some good news, so YOU BE OUR MIRACLE. I did love taps through blown kisses tonight through the window. I told him I would see him tomorrow and he had best be good tonight. We are all excited for his steps... you keep going... do you hear? YOU KEEP GOING! I love you with my heart and soul and I will see you tomorrow.

Quick 6 pm update. Mike did well with his turns. Endured well. He has hung in steady. Thank you, God.

Mike, God, his wonderful medical team, and our prayers have given us a few baby steps to grasp on to.

Individual prayer requests:

For complete healing and home to us.

For calmness but a fight for Mike.

For prevention and control of secondary infection.

May his lungs continue to 'pop' may his oxygen levels get better may Mike be these workers well-deserved success miracle story.

Love, Sarah

Quotes: "If you wish to move mountains tomorrow, you must start by lifting stones today."

"You have been assigned this mountain to show others it can be moved."

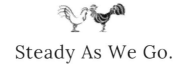

Steady As We Go.

"At the end of the day, all you need is faith and strength. Faith that it will get better, and strength to hold on until it does."

As always:

Beat the bumps.

God is more powerful than covid.

#Keepthelightsonformikey

Steady as we go.

Scripture: "But if we hope for what we do not see, we wait for it with patience." Romans 8:25

Reflection: "When people patiently and expectantly wait on God amid horrible circumstances, suddenly God breaks through. So, don't give up. Don't stop believing. Stay full of hope and expectation. God's power is limitless, and He'll break through for you." -Joyce Meyer-

PRAY

Day 29 / May 6

I want to thank everyone for continuing to support me, our kids, and our families throughout this. The people rooting and praying for Mike is just the most amazing thing. It is overwhelming but I believe it is needed and every single person following Mike and praying for him along this road is working. One last article has been written to tell of Mike's story, COVID, vaccines, and health care today by our old hometown paper, The Haldimand Press. It was an excellent article, one for which I appreciate more awareness going into the community. I don't think you might find another person with more of a love of Haldimand Norfolk than Mike....I think that when he is well, he will run for mayor. He has always thought this is just the best place in the world to live. When we first started dating, I had just come back from living in Lake Louise and was a little bit in love with life out there. Not that Mike did not love me but when I mentioned moving back out west, I realized that his love of this community was all-consuming... there is no home for him but here. I loved him more than a mountain and this is where we built our lives. I would not change a moment. Mike is a hometown boy, born and raised, with good values, honest, kind, respects elders, knows how to have a good time, and knows that family is the first thing in life.

So here is what I learned about my Mikey, your Mike, your Chicken today. When I did my early morning call to nurse Jen, I was told he had a solid night. Uneventful. He held his own very well in the night and gave the nurses no trouble. I called at 11.

Steady As We Go.

Tatiana is Mikes' Day nurse today... they know he can hear them as he can acknowledge their presence... she says he is just so weak. He can acknowledge for a minute then so tired. Otherwise holding good. I am unsure whether it will be a room or a phone visit, but I can see him either way.

When I arrive, I wait for a bit while they change his dialysis filter. They finish early and tell me that I can come in. Great news I can go in the room! They have moved his roommate and I can see him. Tatiana goes over his info... he is holding steady. Oxygen on the EMCO, and vent the same, no bleeding, sedation they are trying to lower. Baby steps being answered.

I gowned up and went in to see my Mikey, to see his eyes open... his eyes were open!! I went to his bedside and said Hi Mike, it's me, it's Sarah, I love you so much. I know you can see me; I know you can hear me. I am so happy to see you. His breathing became a bit labored then, his hands started moving, he was trying to tell me he knows I am there. Tatiana quickly comes in. They don't want to sedate him, they want him to learn how to work through this so as she in her calming voice telling him not to be scared, to breathe, breathe Mike. I was scared. I didn't know whether to tell him to breathe faster or breathe slower, so I just started. You gotta know when to hold them, know when to fold them, know when to walk away, know when to run... you never count your money when you are sitting at the table there will be time enough for counting when the dealings done (I have no answer for why I keep doing this or singing, I think I get comfort from how I have watched that song bring so much happiness to Mike... so that is my answer). Between the two of us, most definitely Tatiana, the breathing Mike got under control. It was such a love to see his eyes. I know they saw me. I can physically see the work he is doing. His body and mind and strength-giving everything he has. I probably repeat myself over and over, but I told him he could rest his eyes I know he is there and listening, but he kept them open for 15 minutes and then on and off glimpses. I told him his reasons to live. His loves, his friends, his farming life, his family. That certain Ireland Road people are driving down at 5 in the morning to touch his wall and say hurry your ass back. I prayed for him and while I did, the bed beside was being cleaned by the wonderful people that make sure everything is disinfected to the highest degree, as I said Amen. Rosie as I know her name, looked at me and said, "Amen."

I did some sports updates, I sang, reinforced his need to be here for his kids. We must move Zack to Brock next year, Ryan will hopefully have his OHL camp in Flint. Mike this was just as much your dream as Ryan's. Alexis needs her 'brotha.' She is so talented too and who knows, she is so determined she will get whatever she wants in life. Holly who needs you for grade 9 and is as you would want her to be doing. She is contacting schools for hockey because she is living what you have always ingrained in all our kids. Mikey. This is all your doing.

    I sang a bit more, then said I had to go. I know you are tired but here is the deal. You rest when you can but when they ask you to work... YOU WORK.

    Tatiana says he is doing very well for where we stand right now, she is proud of him. I gave Mike his love taps...I don't even tell him how many friends he has anymore, as my

Steady As We Go.

one reporter friend said, "He will need a press conference when he gets out of here."

Specific prayers:

May, his lungs continue to pop.

May he be returned to us completely healed.

May, the levels of sedation, calmness awareness all be balanced.

May, Mike, not be afraid. May he feel and be led towards healing.

Quotes:

"God says, Stay patient. My timing is perfect. I have something bigger planned for you, and trust me, you're going to love it."

"Deep inside of you is more strength than you have ever known."

"Our prayers may be awkward. Our attempts may be feeble. But since the power of prayer is in the One who hears it and not in the one that says it, our prayers do make a difference."

"In our waiting God is working!"

As always:

#Keepthelightson

more baby steps my Mikey

beat the bumps.

steady as we go.

Love, Sarah

Scripture:

Matthew 7:7 "Ask, and it will be given to you seek, and you will find, knock and it will be opened to you".

Reflection:

"When we take the time to pray, we acknowledge our dependence upon the Lord and His grace and mercy. We can't fight our battles without Him. God doesn't need your prayers because He knows exactly what you need before you even ask, but we need Him in our lives so desperately." Author Unknown.

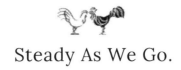

Steady As We Go.

CALM

Day 30 / May 7

Day 30... I can't believe that we have come this long or this far. But Mike has come this far, he has survived this long, he has beaten the odds on more than one occasion, and he has defied them. I am so proud of him. I am, his kids are, his family, his friends. My heart bursts for him. It is like a mom or dad watching your child take their first step, their first word, their first hug... it is the baby steps. He is doing right now what he needs to do. For those who don't know Mike, I always try to share a memory of the kind of guy that Mike is...those that know him know that Mike does not have an organized wallet... in fact it is atrocious. Who goes to the hospital with $200 cash in it? Mike's wallet is the source of many searches. He is never overly concerned. His wallet (and phone) has been left at the Simcoe Arms over night... only to have Lynda or Mary -Ann answer his phone calls. His wallet has been found on fence posts throughout our farm. His wallet has countless times been kicked across the dust of a ball diamond in his anger. My favorite, we have had his wallet Purolator-ed home from the Don Cherry's in Niagara Falls, that one was a treat. But I guess I am sayin, Mike is busy living, he is never worrying or bothering, and I want that to be your focus. Live, love, hug, wrap your arms around your person. Smell their smell... and breathe it in. This is what I learned today about my Mikey, your Mike your Chicken.

Stephanie was his evening nurse and she said he had a steady rock-solid night prayer answered.

I did not get a hold of his day nurse till noon. Andre is his nurse today. I can go at 3 again today. I am once again so excited to see Mike. I go up and gown up and go in to see Mikey. His eyes are open again! Hi my Mikey. I love you, hi, I now know how to read the heart monitor, so I watch it to see and now learned I want a low heart rate so I talk to him calmly. Andre came in. I've got to say, I love for Mike to have a male nurse. He talks to him like a guy you must be tough, you are a superhero, you are doing so good, you keep fighting, you keep up the good work. Mike's x-rays show improvement, his numbers remain the same. Sedation is lessened. This is Mike's uncomfortable stage. He will be uncomfortable. We need to get him to the next stage. Truly the keyword is "breathe," so I share with you now.

Breathe in love and breathe out fear. Breathe in peace and breathe out stress. Breathe... slowly. Gently... deeply...

Just Breathe. Dr. Ainsworth came into the room to talk to me, an amazing man. the same man I met with Sunday to tell me that Mike was against a wall, he had no room and now he has a little bit of breathing room... HE IS FIGHTING.

I continued to talk to Mike. I prayed for Mike and all that he stands in need of. I prayed for calm, I prayed for understanding for Mike, for the power of prayer, that he be protected from any other forces.

I am going to end with one more thing, today I received a message. I do from many people in a day. This was from a man, I do not know him, but his message was this. I have read about you on the HHS website, I know of your husband's case and that he is on ECMO. I have a dear friend

Steady As We Go.

who is in the same hospital and was placed on ECMO yesterday. I am hoping to follow your story. You are so encouraging, and we would like to follow you, we are living your life. This is the thing, there are countless people like my Mikey in this hospital, in this province, in this country.

I have chosen to make it vocal. I have made Mike "Our Story." For some reason I can...and I want these prayers for Mike. I believe these prayers are healing him and lifting him up. There are countless people out there living our story, they just didn't choose our platform. As well as praying for my Mike tonight may we pray for an end to Covid and everyone's suffering. May we continue to lift these health care workers, these super people. They are. I honestly don't have words to say what they mean to me.

Individual prayers:

Ultimate (earthly) healing for Mike.

May, his lungs continue to pop.

Secondary infections be kept at bay.

Pray for peace for Mike and fight when needed.

Quotes tonight:

"Every miracle in the bible started as a problem."

"Take the first steps. Then another. It always seems impossible until it is done."

"The Lord himself will fight for you. Just stay calm, difficult roads often lead to beautiful destinations."

"Put on your full armour of God."

As always:

Baby steps my Mikey.

#Lightsonformike

Steady as we go.

Love, Sarah

Scripture: "The Lord himself will fight for you. Just stay calm." Exodus 14:14

Reflection: God can calm the storms in your life and in your heart. Despite your fears, God can fill you with his peace.

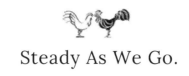

Steady As We Go.

BREATHE –TAKE 2

Day 31/ May 8

Today it has been one month since I dropped Mike at the doors of the NGH, hoping that what I suspected was true was not. Hoping that when he texted me that he had Covid and would be in the hospital for a few days, that it was true. Praying that he would be back home a few days later, all better and ready to go. God sometimes has a different plan than what we think he should or basically what we want of him. I am not going to lie. I hate this plan. I hate every single second of what is happening. I hate what I feel, I hate what our kids and our families feel, and I hate what our friends are feeling. But I know as much as I struggle with it that God knows how we already feel. His heart hurts with ours, Am I angry? Am I sad? I am, but I know that all things are possible with prayer and God, and I take comfort in knowing that he wants to be asked, so this is what we do… we pray because God is capable of anything which I believe, and Mike believes. To think that a whole month has gone by. It is unfathomable… yet life is still going by, and Mike would want that. If this were your loved one in this situation, he would be bringing you by a beer in the laneway just to make sure you were ok. He would be a cheerleader for you. Mike loves his friends with a passion, they are more than friends. They are family. I appreciate the family that I have today. But I have a lot of info today, so enough about Mike. He hates attention anyway; he has a lot he is going to have to get over.

This is what I learned about my Mikey, your Mike your Chicken today. At 5:30 this morning I started off with a particularly good report from night nurse Stephanie (I honestly believe her voice could soothe anyone). Mike had a great last night. She lightened his sedation. His DC-ECMO, settings are down a bit. They tried him on a setting where he had to do the work on his own for a bit and he did! My heart just swells with love and pride. I just want to jump on him and hug him so tightly. They did increase sedation for a bit which was a well-deserved break... Stephanie asked how I am doing. We talked for a bit. I look forward to her being Mike's nurse again.

Today Andre again. Spoke to him at 11. Mike was very aware when he started his shift. All is the same... simply trying to walk him through this, calm breath. See you at 3 Andre. When I arrived at 3, I gowned up to see Andre doing his charting inside the room so that he can talk to Mike... be still my heart. Mike is fighting the fight of his life. His ECMO settings are down. Andre said to Mike, "Mike you are doing so much better than you are feeling, just keep fighting and working". Mike was awake the whole time... off quite a bit of sedation, although it would be easy to give him more... this is the best way to get him through this... must go through this to get to the next phase. He is nailing it. The DR. came in, who one week ago said Mike was up against a wall, he today came in and gave me a thumbs up and said he is leapfrogging... He is by no means counting Mike out of the woods yet, but he is so impressed with his work ethic over these 48 hours... he was put in a corner and the athlete/ English award winner/ you ain't cheatin if you ain't tryin guy is coming out to battle. Mikey needs to be resilient and calm

Steady As We Go.

and focus on his breathing. I told him each hour will get better and better, each day Mikey... you must keep going, keep fighting. Do not quit. Do not go anywhere but towards your family and friends. I did the usual today. But now calming is the utmost important job. There is no room for my tears. Save them for another day. He must see happy eyes. It takes a bit to get breathing back in control. Honestly slow... calm... slow ... calm... (I'm honestly not sure my singing does that, so I am using "apple music," way more). I told him all the news at home always saying Mikey I can't tell you this if you can't slow your breathing... anyway we all know what I said. Love, prayer. Always I pray for Mike when I get there, before I leave, videos. I can see the reaction now; he can see and hear. Love not being tired. Focus on memories and I talk about what is to come. I told him don't worry my, Mikey I am getting good at these one-sided conversations. I am sure you have so many contradictions to what I am saying but too bad. Listen and learn.

Oh my, I could go on and on but as you know Mike is my cause, so I leave you with this. Yes, Mike has leapfrogged... yes, I can see his eyes, but I will say Mike is still fighting because now he faces the pain portion in weaning him towards being off machines. Yes, this is a process and yes this is best for him... he is on pain medication too, but to reach the next step, we need to limit sedation. Mike has lived through pain before. I am believing he will once again conquer.

Long post I know... one more shout out to these workers... who, where would we be without them? Andre and

I talked for a few minutes when I left Mike's room. He was headed back to clean Mikey up and talk sports to him. This is a debt Mike, nor I will ever be able to repay. We head into Nurse's week. Do you know one? If you do, please say thanks.

Individual Prayer Requests:

A complete Covid healing, keeping from secondary concern.

I pray for calm for Mike... may he breathe through this anxiety and pain.

Pray for this brilliant medical team. From the floor cleaner to the gown washers to the doctors and nurses and my ECMO man.

Continue the miracle prayer.
Quotes:

"Success is the sum of small effort repeated day in and day out."

"You're off to great places! Today is your day! Your mountain is waiting, so get on your way." (For you Mike)

"Every single time my heart beats and my lungs expand, God is telling me "Keep living I am not finished with you yet".

As always:

Beat the bumps my Mikey.

Breathe Mikey, breathe.

Steady as we go.

Love, Sarah

Steady As We Go.

Scripture: Matthew 6:34 "Sometimes we need to be reminded to breathe, just breathe and be, just be. Not to worry about tomorrow for tomorrow will bring its own worries but just be and live in the moment."

Reflection:

It is GOD who breathes life into us. We all need to take a deep breath and truly breathe in the Holy Spirit.

Jesus, we ask you to breathe new breath into Mike. Continue to work on healing those lungs and to walk alongside him in his fight. Keep him calm and relaxed and able to feel and inhale your presence. We know you have this. We praise you and we trust you and we love you. Amen.

RESCUE

Day 32 / May 9th

Today is a couple of special days. It is Mother's Day which I would truly rather forget but I realize both Mike and I have great friends who are Moms. I have a great Mom; Mike had a wonderful Mom as well. Today is the first Mother's Day Mike and I, his brother Kevin, and his wife Cindy, and their dad Jack do not have her here with us, so I am struggling taking any well wishes this year for Mothers Day.

What I would rather talk about is that this is National Nurses Week. This is something that brings a smile to my eyes. I am passionate about this week. My life has been changed by these people and my husband has received life saving care. This building, this hospital is an institution and although it is nurses week, it takes everyone from the screener inside the door, the cafeteria worker, to the floor cleaner, to the people that are sterilizing the rooms... it takes every single person to ensure this building is the safest place it can be for it's patients and every worker inside. From the person who answers this phone when I call ICU, to the random mover of medical equipment I encounter. You are important. Work is something we all do to make money... so we can all do the other things we love in life, whatever that may be for you. Work can feel like a transaction... a negotiation of our time to receive our paycheck... our money. Let me tell you that nurses, doctors, health care providers are not transactional ... they are transformational. It is more than a paycheck... it is a purpose. These people are putting their hearts into their work and God sees it. These doctors, and nurses are between the lines of their job description. This

Steady As We Go.

is what sets them apart. Their job description is a set of criteria. What they do between those lines makes them to me the absolute most amazing spectacular people in the world. These are people of transformation. I love them, I have such a respect, an admiration for them, an awe. Be amazed by them. Thank them, love them.

So, this is what I learned about my Mikey, your Mike, your Chicken today. My call this morning, Shannon was Mike's night nurse last night. She was happy with Mike. His sedation is low. She is hopeful for how his night went. Thank you so much Shannon. Enjoy your days off and thank you for your care.

Today's day nurse is Chris... another male nurse who I just think is awesome! They are amazing and I am so happy that Mike has these men to care for him. I say this in no disrespect, but I think Chris's voice could lull anyone to sleep so if you want Mike to be calm. I think this is our guy. Chris in his very calm voice told me this morning that it is their hope today to get Mike off dialysis... they also hope to get him off ECMO...today. Pardon Chris? Did I mishear your calm soothing voice? I did not... that is the plan. THANK YOU, GOD. His gases are perfect, he is doing good, Mike is anxious... so nurse Chris has changed his anxiety medicine a bit. Chris knows he is scared and wants to help with it. See you at 3 Chris.

When I arrived in ICU, I was met by this lady coming straight at me... all business, I did not recognize her, but she got straight to work... do you know what is going on with Mike? I read her nametag quickly.

Connie, perfusionist (ECMO lady). I get so caught up in my ECMO man's eyes that I didn't know I had a woman too. She tells me this... (I tell you this with reserved hesitation because Mike needs prayers for this to work, for him to be lifted. In my heart I would like to wait until it is accomplished to tell you, but I can't because I believe in you all and the power of prayer and I believe if I want it prayed for. I need to ask you to join me). I would like to update only tomorrow at noon and say it is done, but I have taken you through every step, from bleeding urine, to blood pressure, to oozing sights. I will take you here too. As of 1:27 this afternoon Mike has been capped from his ECMO machine. It is still there but is doing no work. Mike and his vent are working together, but his vent is on good settings. He needs to be good for 12 hours on this and tomorrow, God willing, the ECMO will be removed.

Mike needs to be calm over these hours. Pray for calmness and God's peace for Mike now and in this process. After Connie told me this, all gowned up I hugged my cousin as a nurse on this floor, I hugged her for all I had, for hope, for their work, for their dedication, for My Mikey. I hugged and I held on... Thank you Connie. My ECMO lady.

My visit with Mike. Chris was in the room with him. Mike is calmer today. They have administered a tad of sedation to calm him. His vent is doing some of the work, but Mike is doing a lot of the work, so they don't want him being overly anxious.

While I was in with Mike, another huge thing is that they took him off dialysis. What a day. I knew they could

Steady As We Go.

possibly, but they unhooked him while I was there. Mike's eyes were a little more closed today, he is resting. Nurse Chris came in to wake him up and he roused. So many things to say but I want to say two stories quickly... Firstly I can see Mike is more tired today, and as I am talking, I feel like I may be talking to a wall. (Like the old days.) I ask Mike, do you hear me? He nods his head. I LOVE YOU.

One more story. I tell Mike lots of memories, lots of fun times. We go to Turkey Point each year to our cottage for a week and a half. We have quite a crew that goes now. We always try to find activities to do. Two years ago, we decided, well more so our good friends "The Woods", (Woody and Chal) decided, let's go mountain biking through the trails with their buddy Meiklejohn. We loved every single moment. Mike hated every second from the second he entered the path and scraped his knuckles on the trees to every single turn, every uphill pedal, or downhill miss the root path. He hated it and shouted his hate every turn and every moment. His best time was when it was done, and he got his free drink back at the Second Sand Bar. Which he may have drank in record time.

My point is, today I told him that Woody (nickname to our great friend who was with us) told me to tell you about this summer at the cottage. He wants to mountain bike again. Mike's head shook back and forth... NO. Ok, Mike you don't have to. You are hearing.

Wrap up... Dr. Craig came into the room. Same man who a week ago today told me that Mike was against a wall...

he needs to make some steps. The same man who saw me sobbing in front of him comes in today. I know he is smiling under his mask. Be optimistic. Mike is amazing us (he shouldn't amaze you because you are amazing health care people and God, and you are all superheroes.)

I had the same visit with Mike. I talked, prayed, I told him about us all. Today, I showed him videos of our kids, some friends, and our farm. He loves this place. It is his passion, his and Kevin's, taken over from Jack. He knows he is loved. For those that know me, I honestly told him, to suck it up... you be strong... we can be weak when we are home again together so until then suck it up, we can "heal later" together!

I know I am leaving today with a believing heart. I will say it again. I believe in Mike, I always have, I will until the day I die. I believe in the reach he has. The vaccination pictures continue to roll in who otherwise wouldn't, the Covid awareness. Yes, it is real, the awareness of these workers... be amazed be awed. We all know one or two. Say, thanks. You have no idea the trenches they are in. Finally for the power of prayer. I believe, God made extremely smart people like Mike's doctors, his nurses, his ECMO people. I thank him for them. But I also believe in what these thousands have united in is working. God wants to hear people asking him... it is not ego... it is the way it is. He already knows what we want. Just keep asking. Mike is getting so close to the finish line. Help him to get him across it. May he finish with his swagger, his all-purpose shoes, and may there be a Giant Stella waiting for him.

Individual prayer requests:

Steady As We Go.

We pray for complete healing of Mikey.

Pray for calmness for Mike and clearness of mind.

Pray that Mike succeeds with the ECMO being capped, 12 good hours and off tomorrow with a lifetime of good hours to follow.

Pray for secondary infection to be far, far, away.

Quotes:

"Today's accomplishments were yesterday's impossibilities."

"Use the pain in your past as FUEL. Fuel that will drive you straight to a better future."

"Good things are manifesting."

"Better things are happening."

"BEST things are coming."

Quote: *"In the middle of the darkest night. In the middle of the hardest fight, it's true, I will rescue you."* Lauren Daigle

As always,

Beat the bumps, Mikey.

If you ain't cheatin you ain't tryin.

You've got this my Mike.

Steady as we go.

"Rescue," by Lauren Daigle

Scripture: "I will call on God and the Lord will rescue me." Psalm 55:16

Reflection: Rescue: "to be saved from a distressing situation." As Mike ventures through some difficult days ahead with handling pain and the exhaustion of focussing on breathing, I pray the Lord continues to come to his rescue. Sarah, we pray you continue to tread above water and feel the love of God holding you up-he is also rescuing you.

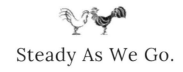

Steady As We Go.

POWERFUL

Day 33 / May 10th

I know everyone knows what a big day this was for Mike... how a lot of things depended on his evening... how he handled being capped from the ECMO. How his night went. When I called down at 5:30 in the morning to talk to nurse Sylvia his night had gone well. He was doing it, using the vent and not the ECMO. Plans remained for the removal of the ports for this morning. If they don't feel they should move him to an operating room, they will turn his room into an operating suite. They will do it.

So, this is what I learned about my Mikey, your Mike, your Chicken today. I thought I understood what it was to wait, to be anxious, to be a little bit of a new level of panic, but once again. I have never been good at waiting, and I proved no better today. Patience is a virtue. At 10:30 I got the most beautiful call from Dr. Craig. Mike is off ECMO. They did it bedside and Dr. Craig said it went super smooth. I could hear the delight in his voice. He did not need to call me... one of the nurses could have, but he called me personally. I love this man. How do you thank someone for saving your someone? The thing is, you don't need to, he is so happy. Helping Mike makes him happy. It's as simple as that. This is what he lives for. I thanked him so much. He said see you this afternoon. I prayed, I clapped, I happy danced around my table. Thank you, God.

My visit is at 3:00 again today. Melissa is Mike's nurse today. When I arrived, Dr. Craig is in room with Mike. He comes out to see me and they are just so pleased. His sites look good. He is doing well. They are optimistic. His eyes are smiling... they should be, you helped my Mikey cross a hurdle. For those that know me I am not a hugger, I hate hugging... for Lent every year when people give things up. I add them. I add to be a better hugger each year, but I tell you, if I could wrap this man in my arms, I would. I gowned up and went into see Mike. He does not have much sedation... the quicker through this phase the better. Mike is so much less tubed. So much weight off his body in equipment. So much less machinery to step through to get to Mike. He is very aware. I know he is scared and anxious, but that is what we need to pray for. I know that he doesn't really know what has happened, but I know that he knows what I am talking about. Basically, right now I am his biggest cheerleader with the most motivational speeches (we will deal with the ego later). I need him. I told him how much he is loved and needed. I showed videos of our kids... therefore you are fighting. Mike had a friend; I think I have mentioned who was in Burlington ... when Mike was there at the same time. Pete came off the vent the day before Mike went on. Pete is home and I tell Mike that I don't know the pain you are in... but I do know that Pete does... and I know he knows you can do it. You can get through. Do not give up you are almost there and then we are going to talk... about this most crazy time we have had. Pete knows... he knows what you are feeling, and he says stick with it.

Just a few more things. I said yesterday how when I came in the hallway of ICU, I was met by this lady coming at me who turned out to be my ECMO- lady for the day saying she had capped Mike off, we had 12 hours... she is focused.

Steady As We Go.

Today the door opened and in comes this lady. I hear you are calling me the ECMO- lady! Yes, I am because that is what you are. She is so happy. But she has a story. ECMO- lady Connie is from Calgary. She got deployed here, went home, came back, and hasn't left. She was supposed to last week, but she got asked to stay again. So, she did. She has a one and six-year-old at home in Calgary, but she knows she is needed here. She loves this staff and Ontario needs her. Mike needs her. She is super brilliant. I said there isn't enough money in the world to repay you. I don't do it for the money. That is what makes you so special. While chatting with her, my ECMO- man comes in the room. Two of my favourite people... We already know that the ECMO- man has amazing eyes and a voice but these two had a success today, so to see them and me chatter for a few minutes. Man, they deserve this success they deserve this they are proud, giddy... a moment of success in a depressing job. ECMO man... woman... my gratitude can never be repaid.

Lastly, I gave Mike his love taps, all my love.

I WILL SEE YOU TOMORROW. I told him I want to stay forever but Mikey I am confident leaving you because these people care like no one else. You are safe and God is watching.

As I was leaving, I saw Dr. Craig in the hall and said thank you for everything... his answer was. "See you tomorrow."

Love, Sarah

Individual prayer requests:

For calm for Mike for easy breathing… breathe in breath out.

Ports to heal.

Ultimate and total healing from Covid, for Mikey.

For the doctors and nurses and the rest of the patients.

Quotes:

"God desires to show his power through your storms."

"Out of the darkness the Lord speaks and instructs us to move forward as he makes a way."

"No matter how tall the mountains it cannot block the sun."

As always:

Baby steps, Mikey.

Let go and let God.

You've got this.

Steady as we go.

Love, Sarah

Scripture: "But I will restore you to health and heal your wounds," declares the Lord. Jeremiah 30:17

Reflection: God, please continue to fill Mike with the healing power of your Spirit. You are a miracle worker, and we see your hard work in the ICU. You are the greatest physician. You are so very present. Please calm him, prod him lovingly and gently and remind him to keep breathing.

Steady As We Go.

Give him confidence in the power of your grace, that even when he is afraid, he can put his whole trust in you. Make him whole and a walking testament to your power. God as you make your rounds-please touch others who are walking down this same difficult road and remind them, that you are more POWERFUL and BIGGER than their storm.

LOVE

Day 34 / May 11th

I want to start by saying how so very, very, proud I am of Mike. He seems to be my all-consuming thought these days. Everything else has gone out the window, I try to be the best mom I can be but otherwise, I can't really concentrate on too much besides praying, making sure my kids are doing the best they can be and focusing all my strength and energy on Mike. I don't say this for anyone to think I need anything. I know I have the best friends; I have a freezer that is packed, I have love, I have rides, I have support. What I need from people who are wondering what they can do for me is this, you continue to do what I have asked all along, you pray for Mike, for complete healing. You pray for these doctors, nurses and all who work within hospital walls... not only Mike's hospital but all hospitals, that these people are ready for the battle.

Mike has always been a talker, he loves telling a story, he loves to have the quick comeback... his voice can always be heard in a room. It draws you in. Then you see his smile. You can never just have one beer... it's always, "Just one more," and I know with all my heart that I am going to have that again, but do I ever miss his voice, just hearing him talk to me. He is so good at making people smile with his words. I can hear his laugh. I'm going to hear it soon... we all will because I am going to tape his first laugh and send it out so you all can know this guy ... this Chicken who I am so happy to be able to call mine.

So, this is what I learned today about my Mikey, your Chicken, your Mike. Sylvia was Mike's night nurse again last

Steady As We Go.

night and she had an uneventful night. Mike has done well off the ECMO. They are happy with him. Mike's day nurse is again Melissa. Dr. Craig is once again back in today and is looking after Mike again today. He is just so skilled and calm. He has a sense of assurance about him, and it is so obvious the respect he has from the nurses, I am sure because he gives respect to them as well. I had my visit with Mikey. Let me tell you, I am just so happy to see him every day. I know I am there to reassure him, but he reassures me, because he keeps fighting. He knows what he must live for.

Mike is working hard...he knows what hard work is about... he lives it every day. Having a farm, having an outside job, having kids who are active in sports every night. This guy is not afraid of the concept of work. Now he is learning to breathe again... with lungs that aren't quite 100 percent yet. It's a labour. It is the part that must be done to be able to move to the next step, but it is hard work, and I can see it in him. I spoke lots to Mike. His brother called and spoke to him on speaker which was good for both. Now, I feel my job is to be "a calmer." Reassure him, love him, share some happy memories with him. I prayed for him... always, for complete healing for thankfulness for another visit, for peace and calm, doctors, and nurse's wisdom, for a fight inside Mike, for the David in Mike to conquer this Goliath. I pray for the surrounding of Mike, for a storming of heaven on his behalf. I talk about the kids, show some videos. Remind him again of all the things that we are going to do... whether it be burn the burn pile because I am too afraid to do that without him or sit on the cottage deck and have a beer... (or just one more) and "people watch." He nods, I know he wants these things too. We asked Mike for steps... in this last week with his back against the wall, he started racing! We are so proud of him. The breathing tube has been in Mike for quite some time now... it is still doing its job, but the longer it's in, the greater source of infection it could be so Dr. Craig has decided that tomorrow morning they will take it out and another excellent Dr will be putting in a tracheotomy. Dr Craig had talked to me days ago about this being a possibility so please don't get your knickers in a knot. I knew this might happen and this is best for Mike. I have a few respiratory therapist friends who have wondered when this would happen. This will give Mike his mouth back, ease his discomfort and as Dr. Craig says this prepares him for the road to his recovery. He needs to gain strength, muscle, and rest. These steps he has taken in the last few days have been huge and exhausting.

So, we trust in God, we trust in these people I have been entrusting Mike to for 34 days and we continue the journey. Mike is confident enough to nod his head and know what he is fighting for, great enough to hold my hand, I see the love in his eyes watching his kids on video. This will help him get there that much faster. Speed has never been Mike's strong point; he gets there when he does... usually with five or six social stops along the way.

I had a chance to visit with ECMO man and ECMO woman tonight, as much as I wish I could say they were out of a job, they are not. Please don't forget this is Nurses Week. They need our gratitude, our love, our thanks. It doesn't look like their workload for their floors is lessening anytime soon. Get a needle, be safe, be aware, pray and thanksgiving.

Love, Sarah

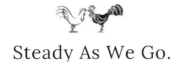

Steady As We Go.

Individual prayer requests:

Pray for complete healing of Mike and all covid patients.

Pray for calm and understanding for Mike.

Pray that the trach goes according to plan and with ease tomorrow.

Please pray for these health care workers.

Quotes: *Philippians 4:6, "Do not be anxious about anything, but in everything, by prayer and petition, with thanksgiving, present your request to God."*

"Behind every scar, there is an untold story of survival."

"The difference between being a stumbling block and a steppingstone is how high you raise your foot."

And this one is totally about Mike…

"I love people who have no idea how wonderful they are and just wander around making the world a better place."

As always:

Beat the bumps Mikey.

Let go and let God.

If you ain't cheatin, you ain't tryin.

Steady as we go.

Quote: *Joshua 24:15, "His love gives life."*

Scripture: Corinthians 13:13 "And now these three remain, faith, hope and love, But the greatest of these is love."

Reflection: God's Love is called AGAPE. It is a Love like no other. Your family. Your friends. Your community. Your new friends in the ICU. Have all given and received love. It is a beautiful thing. But God's unconditional love for you. That Love will be exhausted it will never need a rest and it is there for you even when you don't realize it. Agape love has no limitations.

Love is given. It is felt. Mike's journey has been about these three things. Faith. Hope. Love.

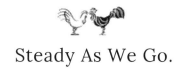

Steady As We Go.

PEACE

Day 35 / Wednesday, May 12

I think of all the ways the world has changed since April 8. We have had snow, we have had trees budding, apple blossoms, grass growing and need to be cut. We have personally shipped a whole crop of chickens that Mike started and for the most part, our son Ryan finished. The fields are being worked, farmers are busy, the days are getting longer. We are heading into one of Mike's favorite times of the year... the land readiness, watching crops sprout. I am careful what I say now to Mike... I don't want him to know how long he has been there. I am sure that would be frightening. I know that he knows he is in the hospital... I am sure he wonders why we are all dressed like we are, but I don't want him to be anxious that he has missed all this time. He would hate that as much as knowing that people are paying attention to him and thinking about him. I want to share two comments friends of ours made last night because it sums up Mike to a tee. The first is from Chad Strohm an old-time ball friend and he said this of Mike..." You said it and I can hear it, 'Just one more', which always means three or four more and another story and one more after that. Great to hear he is on the path back. It reminds me of him at bat. He may have had two strikes but he's fouling them off and fighting back to get one he likes. Working to get the count in his favour... He always comes out on top".

The second from our good friend, Woody who said to me last night, "I look at this as a typical 'Chicken' journey much like the touring of New York. He can only walk so far before needing a break to rehydrate. He's just pit-stopping for a quick refresher to keep moving on to the next stop. Same as Turkey Point or any other venture that guy has ever gone on. 'Quick one', then we can move forward."

So here is what I learned today about my Mikey, your Mike, your Chicken today. Nicole took care of Mike during the night, and he did well. Sedation was lightened, his vent was operating at minimal settings. Trach was still planned for this morning.

Thank you, Nicole.

At about 10:45 I am getting 'antsy' so decide I need to call to see what is happening. Jane is Mike's Day nurse today and she says he is doing excellent. Physio was in this morning, they had him sitting on the side of his bed for a short spell! WOW! She said he was for the most part calm, they planned the trach for noon... roughly, he would be sedated. Jane and I decided to visit at 4. When I arrived, I was a bit nervous (a lot nervous), but I was met by a smiling eyes Jane. Everything went great, smooth, he is ok, sedation still evident but weaning now. Trach looks good!!

Thank you, Jane.

Quick lesson because I had no idea. A trach is still hooked up to a vent, it just uses a neck port as opposed to a whole tube down your mouth and throat. It is less invasive, more comfortable, more versatile for the patient. It gives this option; he can use the vent but also the vent can be removed from the trach connection and the hi flow oxygen can be hooked up to see how he responds on that. (I had no idea, and

Steady As We Go.

I hope my medical expert friends feel I did a good kindergarten explanation of how I think it works).

    I gowned up and went in to see Mike. He looks so much more comfortable than yesterday… the trach is not scary… less so than the tube down his throat, and I can see his cheeks again. His eyes are open. He is not as responsive today, but he had another surgery so… yes you can rest. His hands moved and his eyes opened and closed. He watched some videos.

    I prayed… big prayers of thankfulness, and healing and continued love until Mike is home. Be with these workers, these other patients. So many stories on this floor. Dr. Craig gowned up and came in. Mike has a journey to go, but how do you look at the man who has done so much to save the life of the person you love most in the world… Where do you start? You start with thanks. Dr. Craig is well pleased with Mike, his eyes smile. He says to me… I am going to push him hard; I will not be easy on him; he is going to work. Totally fine Dr. Craig, you push him as hard as you want. You continue to move him through these stages. You are respected by so many; you have a gift; you are doing the job you should be doing. Dr. Craig squeezed my shoulder and said see you tomorrow. My time is up, Mike is tired. His respiratory therapist comes in and explains how she will now stop the vent and put on the hi flow oxygen, and he is doing it, they are pleased.

    I give Mike a last prayer, I give him his love taps, see you tomorrow, Mike. I love you!

In the hall, I truly feel these people are now my friends, I chat with nurse Dianne who says, "Mike has this," because he is Dutch and a farmer! She believes in him. I talked to ECMO-lady, Connie who is so proud of him. I say goodbye to nurse Jane and thank her for taking such good care of Mike and I wave down the hall to ECMO-man who is waving at me. Could there be a more worthy week than Nurses week? 35 days ago, I might have thought there could be... but my eyes are opened in a way I never want yours to be. Angels in scrubs I can assure you.

Individual prayer requests:

For complete healing of Mike's lungs and body, may, Mike remains calm, anxiety low.

Please pray for strength for Mike's physio and for a quick but long enough stay on the track.

Continue to pray for these medical professionals and all staff within these walls.

Pray for the man beside Mike, for the two in the room adjoining for all the rooms that I can't even see.

Quotes:

"Think positive."

"Talk positive."

"Feel positive."

"Start by doing what is necessary; then do what is possible; and suddenly you are doing the impossible."

Steady As We Go.

"The phrase "do not be afraid" is written in the bible over 365 times. That's a daily reminder from God to live every day being fearless."

"The storm that was sent to break you, is going to be the storm that God uses to make you."

As always:

Let go and let God.

Baby steps Mikey.

If you ain't cheatin you ain't tryin.

Steady as we go.

Love, Sarah

Scripture: "Peace I leave with you; my peace I give you. I do not give to you as the world gives. Do not let your hearts be troubled and do not be afraid." John 14:27

God is not a God of disorder, but of peace." 1 Corinthians 14:33

Reflection:

Jesus is the Prince of Peace. Jesus, we ask that you give Mike peace. That you take away his anxiety and fear. That you help him to keep his eyes on you. God. You are his peace. May he see it, hear it, feel it.

Author Sarah VanNetten

RESILIENCE AND PERSEVERANCE

Day 36/ May 13ᵗʰ

I am not going to say that I don't miss Mike. I miss him with everything I have. All the memories I share with Mike... all the stories I tell him, they are reminders because I know he knows what he has at home. We have a good life, we laugh together, we love each other, we compliment each other. He honestly is my better half and the fun parent. Mike has made leaps and bounds these past few days, I am so, so proud of him. I think it was summed up best last night, by friends who basically said when the going gets tough the tough get going. That's Mikey. Anyway, I have a lot to share tonight with you so here goes.

This is what I learned today about my Mikey, your Mike, your Chicken. Mike had a pretty good night last night. They are happy with his oxygen, sedation. They are pleased... thank you again nurse Nicole. Today Mike has nurse Jane again and she is excellent. (I am sure everyone is catching the common theme in the health care workers, and they are amazing) Mike is doing well, monitored on pain. 3 o clock is good for a visit.

When I arrive and am allowed into ICU, I am greeted by the desk nurse and by my other nurse friend. Mike has moved rooms (I knew this would happen but was unsure when) Mike is Covid negative so is moving ICU units. He is just moving down the hall but nonetheless... he is moved, I found my way from my friend to Mikes' new room. He is now in ICU Covid recovery. He has a window bed. He has a ,

Steady As We Go.

"steady as we go" sticker in his window and the pictures the kids sent him. Let me tell you how proud I am of him... you don't imagine the leaps and bounds he has done... even sometimes I struggle to understand. But I see his effort, I see his labor. For us who know Mike... I say this because I know he will recover... but what it does to the lungs... the breathing, the effort, the full-fledged effort. A strong man who has rounded the turn to come back but is now having to do these days. I will never understand this virus. I don't want to. How it has taken the time from my most important people. I don't understand. What I do know is I see Mike in there. I see him in his head nods, his hand holds, and his acknowledgments... this is a man. Fueled, by God led by prayer, through the most powerful medical team I have ever seen who is winning...They are winning!

Today I saw Mike with only a mask on, no gowning up. He was tired. Today they got him to sit on the side of his bed and then they used a lift to get him into a chair. He stayed there for two hours! I am so proud of him... but never doubt Mikey. For those who know Chicken, this is what this does to you... it's real. These are our baby Chicken steps and I have no doubt by next summer he will be sipping a beer in the beer gardens with you.

Mike was tired for my visit. But he worked to keep his eyes open. Mine are just so happy with him. He has new signs in his new window, so people know where he is. Dr. Craig stopped by two times. I could talk forever about this man who has his own family at home but chooses to live with this work family and his patients. I feel in another world we could be good friends… well maybe not as he is saving people's lives and I am just praising him.

Ok, I am blubbering tonight because I honestly am overwhelmed… by Mike… my love for him. His response when he needed to come to bat. I am overwhelmed by these people… you people who many I have never met and have joined us. I am overwhelmed by walking in that hospital every day and seeing what is happening. Mike left Covid bed 13, someone else is in there. These nurses and doctors are not seeing family and grandchildren… they are knee-deep in Covid. Yet they care for ours… and put to the side their own. They are selfless. I will be honest, I never thought I would be here. You have Covid… where did you get it? Not a question here… What can we do to help you?

For me, I feel like "Nurses week", is for the rest of my life. I don't want anyone to walk in my shoes. Nursing is an outstanding career… outstanding and needed. Beyond appreciated.

Individual prayer requests:

For Mike's lungs to continue popping and healing. For calmness and peace of mind for all patients on the floor.

I pray that medical professionals with days off can have a restful and rejuvenating time with their family.

Quotes:

"Being a few steps behind doesn't necessarily mean failure. Sometimes God is preparing you for a great launch."

"The greatest glory in living lies not, in never failing but in rising every time we fall."

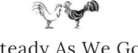

Steady As We Go.

"Failure will never overtake me if my determination to succeed is strong enough."

As always:

Let go and let God.

Baby steps Mikey.

If you ain't cheatin you ain't trying!

Steady as we go.

Love, Sarah

Scripture: Galatians 6:9: "Let us not become weary in doing good, for at the proper time we will reap a harvest if we do not give up."

Reflection: Resilience is the capacity to recover from difficulties. When we face trials, it develops our perseverance. Perseverance is one of the qualities that keeps us productive and purposeful in Christ.

When life throws a punch, it provides an opportunity for spiritual growth. The punch may be hard, but we can trust that God will give the ability to get back up and start again. Robust resilience encourages us to live to fight another day. When life knocks you down, get up. The Lord is upholding your hand. When we find our calmness amid our battles, we become a sanctuary for those battling along side us.

BLESSED

Day 37 / May 14th

Another Friday, another weekend is upon us. Back in the "good old days," I worked out with a group of ladies who are now my friends and now I look forward to Fridays because I know since we can't work out together, our amazing friend, Sue sends us a playlist for the week... always well thought out, appropriate, with a mix of fun, love, worship, and its work time music. Songs are tough to listen to. How do songs evoke such emotion? But I love it I love hearing these songs, their words meaning something. I want to say that yesterday when I left the hospital and was driving home from my ride to the hospital... I listen to county 104, which I love... I heard a song come on I have never heard before and I pretty much had to pull over. I listened to 'Me Without You', by Tim and the Glory Boys. I have never heard this song before, but I feel it played for a reason. I know lots of people have love stories like Mike and I do... I know I am not the first person to ever be in love and be hurting. But when I heard the words to this song, which I had never heard on this station before... I was. This is our song. Listen to the words, they apply to far more people than me but for me now. Mike listens to our song.

So here is what I learned about my Mikey, your Mike, your Chicken today. When I called down this morning Mike had an uncomfortable night. He was complaining of a headache all night. This is a good thing... Mike is not afraid to move his arms calling his nurses in that he is not comfortable. At 5:30 this morn I learned they wanted to take him for a CT scan. Ok. you do what you need to but once again...anxiousness. Someone said to me, when do you feel you will be in the clear

Steady As We Go.

or feel you can breathe... when Mike can text me good night and good morning. I will feel better then.

I called again at 9. Bonita is his nurse today. Great news! He has an ear infection. ENT is in the room with him now, normally we would take the patient to the clinic. but the clinic is coming to Mike. Thank you, thank you. Bonita said a three o'clock visit is fine.

Mike did not have a comfortable night... yet still, rehab continued today... up and at'er Mikey. This is what I LOVE about these people... Mike had no desire to sit in his chair today, they say he clearly looked at his bed, yet tough love, sit in your chair. Here let me take a picture and send it to Sarah... oh, and wave. He also sat on the side of his bed and balanced a bit on his own. Yes, he had a rough night but thank you for a workday today!

When I arrived, Mike is zonked. I get it... as I said to friends... I am going to have to get easier on the naps when he gets home. But I know now when I am there that he can rest, then I need to say, hey Mikey open your eyes, let's talk for a minute... or to be honest the one minute (because I talk to myself all the time now) I am at the window talking about all the pictures that are taped there and their meaning and I look back and it's like 'deer in the headlights'. Oh, you are watching me... look at this Mike. Our reasons!! You all know I could talk forever. I prayed. I played music. Mike got a new roommate today so I was unsure how singing would go but I sing with the Apple music be sure. I tell him how beautiful he is. I tell him of the happenings. I shared the memory of my

40th birthday party of a coach bus trip to Niagara on the lake for a bicycle wine tour that he and Rachel planned, and I said we need to do this again and he nodded. Today Mike is getting good at acknowledging his pain. I can see it in his eyes. So can his nurses and they are good at it... the first-time Mike is just hot... so they put cold clothes on his head... The second I will be honest, he slid his left leg off the bed about 5 times, 5 times I went over and picked it up and put it back on the bed... on time 6 ... I said, well, I guess that is where you want it to be, I am not picking it up again for you.

When I called the nurse the second time for him, she determined his pain was in his hip. so maybe you are dropping your leg and me putting it back up. not a coincidence and you probably wished five times before I would leave your leg alone.

Ok enough tonight... well a few more things... this is a text I received from a friend of our who is known as French guy... he and his wife, Lynn know loss. He texts me tonight and says, "He's a farmer. Farmers never stop working, 24-7, 365 days of the year. The battle he is facing is like, his fields got flooded, and his tractor broke down... but my good old buddy, the way I know him, will only be stronger after this. Chicken guy will drain the fields that are flooded and will fix the tractor and get the work done and will have the best crop after it is all said and done... He will be back home with his family, the best crop a farmer can have."

When I left Mike after I knew he was getting medicine, he was calmer. I prayed again and I love tapped him. See you tomorrow. I got thinking about all these endless hours so I am excited to tell you that tomorrow (thank you Chris and Alida) I am taking in an iPad in which he can watch TSN 24-7 if he chooses. It's his life, his desire... at home he could

Steady As We Go.

watch "Jays in 30" about four times in a row so I don't think he will be bored. I know he wants to be home. I know he is working like none of us have known Mike to work before.

This is my cousin, Chris, very smart lady it turns out, "Now we have to turn to determination and 'NO' is not an option; a brief compromise is the solution."

I leave you with this... tonight, we have an iPad ready to go to Mike tomorrow. So he can watch sports 24-7. He needs something to do. He is restless... he is working. so, while he works, he can watch what he loves. he can watch his Jays, his Leafs. It will be so good for him, and I am so happy. His Leafs made the playoffs!! He deserves to watch them on their way to the cup!

Individual prayer requests:

Pray for Mike's ear infection that the pain may be controlled and healed pray for ultimate and complete healing.

Pray for Mike's calmness and peace yet with the will to tell the nurses when he is uncomfortable.

Pray for the doctors, the nurses and anyone lying in a bed.

Quotes: *"For nothing is impossible with God." Luke 1:37*

"God's grace is not the light at the end of the tunnel, it's the light that guides us through it."

"There are 3 choices in life: give up, give in or give it all you've got."

"When you feel like you are drowning in life, don't worry-your lifeguard walks on water."

As always beat the bumps Mikey.

Let go and let God.

If you ain't cheatin you ain't tryin.

Steady as we go.

Love, Sarah

Scripture: Job 1:21: Blessed be the name of the Lord.

Reflection:

The sun shining in Mike's window makes one think of blessed. It is easy to put God on the side when life is going well, yet it is also easier to praise him then. Praising God through storms isn't always easy. But spending time with him each day does enable you to withstand the storms of life. There are happy sunny days and there are darker days and we should turn God's blessings back to praise. It is difficult to find blessings on those dark days, but they are there if we really look for them. I pray today-you feel God's blessings.

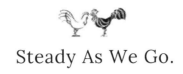

Steady As We Go.

OH, MY HEART...

Day 38: May 15th

I got the chance to speak to J.P. Antonacci, yesterday from the Hamilton Spectator. He had written the article about Mike on May 4th, and he wondered if I could talk to him to update him on how Mike is doing. He has had a lot of people asking and he wants to know himself as well. For sure I will J.P., anything to bring attention to Mike and the causes that he is bringing awareness to. J.P. is so easy to talk to, his questions make sense. He paints Mike to be as he is. He posts pictures that bring out Mike's best features. The article came out today and it was great. I love for people to know the kind of person Mike is, his personality, his love of most things. I love for people to be praying for Mike, thinking about him... understanding what it is like to watch someone you love in this position. To have people picture in their head what it must be like to work on this floor, visit this floor. I am so grateful to have awareness brought to this virus. I honestly think the word virus is too kind for it... this is more than a virus, it is a scary, complicated puzzle that affects each patient differently. These ones who are unfortunate enough to be up here... they are the unlucky ones. For those whom it didn't affect, these people are paying for it 10 000 times over. Virus is not a cruel enough word...I am going to work on a word that is appropriate to sum up the life-changing alterations that it incurs. The first time J.P. called me I told him he would be interviewing Mike himself one day. I told him again today... you will be interviewing Mike yourself someday, and I just can't wait. He said I have no doubt. ...me neither.

So here is what I learned today about my Mikey, your Mike your Chicken. Amy was Mike's night nurse... he had a decent night, some sleep then wide awake, some pain meds, and repeat. She was so great and nice to talk to. She would be calming for Mike. I called back down at 9 am to see how Mike was. Tanya is his nurse today. His ear seems ok. ENT was in to look at his ear. 3 o- clock works for a visit today. I am so excited to get there and bring him the iPad. I thought about it today. His day cannot even be broken up by breakfast, lunch, and supper because there is none... so truly how do you know when one day ends and the next starts?

When I arrived and I look in the room, I can see feet sitting in a chair. Tanya is there and we introduce each other, and I say, he is in his chair? Her response is yes, he is, and he is not happy about it, but I told him he must sit there until you come so he can show you.

I rushed over to his side of the room and there he is sitting up. Mike you are sitting in your chair! You look so amazing and awesome! He puts one hand towards me... the other he uses to bang on his mattress which is right beside his chair. He clearly wants back in the bed. I tell him how proud I am of him. Wow Mikey look at you, you are amazing. BANG, BANG, and looks at the bed. Do you want to go back to bed? He nods. I sit beside him and said, Mike if you want back in our bed then you will sit in this chair and do the work. I pointed at the window with our pictures on it and said those are the reasons you will sit in that chair. I will sit with you and talk to you.

Steady As We Go.

Clearly, he is unhappy with me but has been before. We can save that disagreement for a day down the road. At 3:30 his respiratory therapist came in. She is full of piss and vinegar, and I wish I got her name, but she waves at Mike and does a little sign language thing to him and says to Mike... do you want to show Sarah your trick? Poor guy probably thought no... I want to go back to bed but, he nods yes. They lift him with the lift back into bed which is an amazing machine. While this happens my heart hurts and I say to someone in the room... this was a man full of strength and life 38 days ago and now this is needed. (I know that this is only a step, but to think of the strength and muscle this demon has drained). Mike is comfortable and his RT is by his bed and talking to him and she turns off his vent and attaches another attachment and she says to Mike, "Hi Mike," he whispers back... "Test, test," (this is just her thing, she always does this). Then she says what do you want to say? Mike whispers back, *"I love you."* Mike, I love you with my heart and soul and everything I have. Thank you for saying those words.

Then this love of mine who hates water with a passion because there must be water in beer and chocolate milk, says "I need some water." Break my heart... unfortunately, he is not to the water by mouth stage, but they did reward him with the tiniest ice chip. So hard to see, I can't imagine how dry his throat is. but hopefully soon.

These words-tired Mike right out. But while I am watching him, his right leg slides off the bed and he pulls it back up himself. I said, "Mike! Yesterday I picked your left leg back up 5 times when it dropped. Today you did it yourself!

You are getting stronger. You are." I share with him my texts from his friend Pete who has walked this path to assure him that yes someone knows what you are feeling and what you are feeling is normal, you are winning Mikey. You are! I prayed, I asked him if he wanted me to sing. He shook no. I guess I wasn't as good as I thought. I know Mike is making leaps and bounds. I know he hurts; I know he is sad. I know he is mad. I know he is confused; I have not spoken to him much about the time that has come and gone but this morning when his RT was teaching him the speaking thing, he asked 'what happened?" This breaks my heart, but she explained to him in her peppy voice he had Covid he had some troubles he has fought hard and now he is working to come home.

All in time. I know, but I just want to bring him home today, but I know we have work to do. Today was better than yesterday, hopefully soon he can have that drink, then that meal, then that step then that bath then a walk then a car ride home... but patience for now... for Mike, for me and our family, for us all. He wants it, we are praying for it. Steady as we go for a little while longer in this journey. Once again, I talked to Mike, motivated, or angered him depending on where you sat. I prayed for him. I did not sing but when I left after love taps and my love, he was laying on his side watching Jays in 30 hopefully to nap. Soon my Mikey, you keep working we will pray and keep you coming back to us.

Individual Prayer Requests:

For complete lung healing and return to our home for Mike.

Secondary infections are kept far away.

Steady As We Go.

Pray for patience for Mike and the knowledge to know we must go through this healing for the floor and for people to receive vaccines.

Quotes:

"There are 3 choices in life: give up, give in, or give it all you've got."

"Small steps equal great distances."

"How do you get rid of pain? You don't. You allow yourself to feel it. The body shifts energy for survival. Once you understand it, you make it your friend, so it teaches you a lesson rather than hurts you. Then you grow. Pain is a necessary inconvenience."

As always:

Beat the bumps Mikey.

Let go and let God.

If you ain't cheatin you ain't trying!

Steady as we go!

Love Sarah

Reflection: Lord, I ask that through all this journey, that the eyes of our hearts are opened to see people the way you do. Believe that in difficult times the plaques on our hearts soften and drop off. When our hearts are rendered and torn open by the pain of unforeseeable circumstances, when our hearts are made fertile ground for you to plant your seeds. It is only then, in our pain that we can truly both feel and understand your love for all of us. It is then that we start to grow in you.

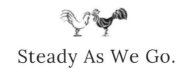

Steady As We Go.

TRANSFORMATION

Day 39 \ May 16th

    This is the time of year I normally call "Lonely farmwife season." For all those farming wives out there, you know exactly what I am talking about. It is the time of year that the field work must be done. Both Mike and his dad would be busy in the fields, Kevin would be delivering seed and the hours would be from sun-up to sundown. An exhausting time of year but one Mike really loves. Many a night picking him up in a field I could barely find. Waiting in the vehicle for the final lap. Passing the time 'tik-tocking' with the girls if they came along for the ride. I must say... I prefer that lonely farmwife season to this. In the future I will never complain about lonely farm wife season ever again. I will welcome it, as it means Mike is home and healthy and sleeping in his own bed and smiling when I bring him supper or a beer and just talking for a minute. It is going to come back, I know it, but farming wives, enjoy this season.

    Today is Sunday, so I listened to church this morning. We all know I believe in God and the power of prayer (working!). But I want to summarize. By no means preach what I learned into a few sentences because this is life lessons. The title was, "Don't Just Sit There." It seemed appropriate for my life right now and Mike... we don't want him to just sit there. This is what I got out of it. We are a society looking for quick fixes to get onto the next thing in our lives. We hurry up to wait, even short waits make us anxious... we don't want to wait...it is our nature now. I think of calling the ICU, the longer I wait online the worse things go through my head and the more places my mind can go. We don't want to wait. Patience is not the ability to wait but the ability to keep a good attitude while we are waiting. Truthfully, some of the things we were in such a hurry for, are turning out to not necessarily be as important as we thought. There is power in numbers. There is power in prayer, as we have witnessed. The act of waiting implies there is something important enough to be waited on, and the waiting for Mike is so worth it. God will go with us each hour of every day. There is no limit to his healing power of whatever healing you or anyone needs, ... mind, body, or spirit. Finally, your most important work is always ahead of you, never behind you....so keep looking forward.

    Here is what I learned today about my Mikey, your Mike, your Chicken. Emily was Mike's night nurse last night. So great to talk to. She has quite a sense of humour. When I called down at 5:30 this morn she was in the room with Mike. She told him I was on the phone, and she was going talk to me. Anything you want me to tell her? He obviously was gesturing with his angry face at his ice chips as when she came to the phone, she said he was doing ok but to tell me she was being mean to him as she was holding back the ice chips he so much wants. I need a smile occasionally. I told her to tell him to suck it up and be a good listener. Thanks for taking such good care of him. I will see him at 3. Day nurse today is Natalie (a different Natalie than before). So many young nurses they have but let me tell you they are all young at heart and have the utmost latest nursing and doctoring techniques. As I walk into ICU, I stop several times so people can tell me how proud they are of Mike, and how are you, Sarah? I talk for a few minutes then get to Mike's room where

Steady As We Go.

he has just freshly gotten into his chair where his physio girls would like him to stay for an hour and a half on the hi flow oxygen. They have big plans and hopes for Mike this week, so he needs to work hard. Perfect, he will do it girls. Mike is so cute. I love him with my heart. He has this thing he does with his hand now... its like a curling of his fingers. Come here it basically says. I go over and sit by him. He is doing much better in the chair today than yesterday, he has yet to pound the mattress. I get the iPad out and we flip between hockey and ball. I tell him how proud we all are, how well he is doing, go over wall pictures again. At about an hour he is looking to his bed. Are you tired? Yes. Ok you just have another half hour to go. Just a look of exasperation and such sad puppy dog eyes. I know you are tired, and he is so wanting water... the reason they are holding back is not to be mean at all, but they do not want it to go in his lungs so for now, he gets a few ice chips and a little sponge because that is what is best for him.

All these years I have been preaching to drink water and now that he wants to, its a no! When he comes home, he will be like I guess water isn't essential after all.

An hour and a half finally pass, and they come to move him to bed. Now I get to see these physio people at work, and they are awesome too! So spunky and direct and just say this is what you must do. I told them I have no problem with tough love and will do whatever you want. As they move Mike into bed, nurse Andre stops by to see him. Mike is a miracle. Miracle helped by prayer. Doctors and nurses like Andre come just to see him and give him his famous line... Mike, I know you don't feel good but trust me you are doing so much better that what you feel! Today's workout, tired Mike, by the time I was leaving he was going to sleep. Good, rest up, be ready for the next workout because you will do this, you will be listening and doing and succeeding. I gave him his love taps and all my love and said I would see him tomorrow. A hockey game was playing on the iPad for him. As I was leaving, I got stopped again with thrilling thoughts of Mike and how well he is doing. Prayers, doctors, nurses, floor cleaners, Mike himself. I believe we are getting there. It is a long road, it will get better each day, don't know anyone more determined than Mike. He is getting stronger every day. I have never seen anyone less afraid of work than Mike. He is on his way from misery to happiness to be Aha, aha, aha, aha, ("I'm on My Way" by The Proclaimers)

Individual prayer requests.

Complete healing for Mike to come home.

Pray for his knee which is currently causing him discomfort (not a big deal but important for when they want to stand him up.)

Pray for these patients' mental health and best thoughts... what they are thinking cannot be easy.

Pray for the doctors and nurses here and in every hospital.

Pray for a removal of covid from our lives.

Quotes

"Maybe life isn't about avoiding the bruises. Maybe it's about collecting the scars to prove we showed up for it."

"Never Give up. Never surrender."

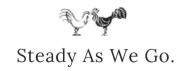

Steady As We Go.

"Rise up."

"Go Beast Mode."

"Never give up."

"And never stop grinding...Period."

As always:

Beat the bumps.

Let go and let God.

If you ain't cheatin you ain't tryin!

Steady as we go.

Love, Sarah

Scripture: Psalm 51:10 "Create in me a clean heart, O God. And renew a steadfast spirit within me."

Reflection: The life cycle of a butterfly is an excellent metaphor for what Mike is experiencing. A caterpillar who crawled into a hospital. Wrapped up in wires and machines in his own chrysalis for a long time. When a butterfly emerges, it takes a while. It needs to gain strength to break through the walls of the chrysalis and time to dry out it's wings before it is to ready to fly. This is Mike. Gaining strength slowly. Soon he will be able to fly. (Yes, this Chicken will fly!) The same God who can move the mountains moves through us and transforms us, not just physically, but spiritually.

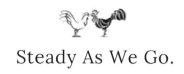

Steady As We Go.

STEADY AS WE GO

Day 40 / May 17th

Day 40... 40 days of life kinda feeling like it has just stopped. 40 days. I find it unfathomable that this is even happening. I honestly don't think I could even talk about it or share this anymore if I didn't believe Mike's progress, his steps forward, his determination is going to be this miracle story we are all praying and rooting for. Mike is such a hockey guy. He lives and breathes it. He has been a coach of all our kids. We have put our full energy into their hockey because they have loved it and have done well at it. We don't vacation, we hockey, and our vacations are spent with hockey families at tournaments and in hallway parties, and neither of us would change a thing. He is so passionate about our kids and going over plays and games and he knows more people in the hockey industry than anyone I know. Everyone loves him. Past people Mike has coached with, kids he taught to skate, kids he has spoken words of encouragement and determination, they can all still hear his words to them. He has often been known to get "fired up" during a game or two while coaching and would come home and say, Sarah, I left the game a little early tonight, the ref didn't see it the way I did and I'm out for a bit. Oh, Mike. Why can't you just keep your mouth shut? But always I heard from everyone else. oh, Chicken was so right, he didn't deserve that. Always on the kid's side. Passionate.

He loves the Leafs! Such a huge fan and I can only hope by the time they win the cup he is home watching the final game on his own couch. Maybe he can be the parade marshal this year. With Mike's sense of humor and smile, he would have the whole team wrapped around his finger in minutes.

So here is what I learned today about my Mikey, your Mike, your Chicken, today. I spoke to nurse Emily this morning about Mike's night, and he had a restful night, the best she has seen him have. Perfect, he is not complaining about much pain, he seems to be ok. Thank you, Emily.

Today Mike has nurse Natalie again, but Natalie and Esther are working their room together. Esther is an OR nurse from Grimsby but because there are no surgeries there, she has been redeployed. She is jumping into a hospital doing a job she knows in an unfamiliar environment, and she is doing amazing. We have two different cases in Mike's room. Bed 1 is an ill patient who although he is not moving, requires so much constant monitoring and discussion, and you have Mike in bed 2 who is a different kind of ill... an active ill, he requires a lot of attention, constant helping to his needs, figuring out what he is trying to say, working with physio, moving him, helping him. I did not see these two ladies rest, I didn't see them complain and every time Mike needed them, they were there with a hop in their step.

Mike was in his chair when I arrived. A different chair today, more a recliner style. Every day he looks a bit stronger, and I tell him. During telling him what a great job he is doing, how many people are thinking of him, I think I must have pulled the up and down handle on the chair to move his legs from kicked out position to hanging down position about 20 times in 20 minutes. I brought him a hockey pool he is

Steady As We Go.

entered in, told him his picks and that he owes his buddy $25. I told him he would be updated every couple of days.

I brought the "Toronto Sun," to read to Mike today. We went over the sports section, and I read him some headlines. I turned on the iPad to replay last night's hockey game. I am telling him what a great job he is doing, and how proud I am of him. He goes between being angry and being frustrated. I told him I know you don't know, but Mike, I watched you in a bed for so long doing nothing, I can come here every day and watch you do something, and you can be mad at me. but choose to use your hour with me wisely... because I miss you. This chair turned out not to be the solution as vinyl is slippery and Mike was sliding down it trying to keep himself up, but we needed physio and they decided to put him back in his bed. Amazing crew here at the Hamilton General Hospital. She said, "Mike you will never see this chair again. While she is there she says to Mike, "I am going to share some exciting news with you. Tomorrow you are going to stand, you are strong enough, I know you can do it. You are going to stand. So, I want you to mentally prepare for it, rest, make your brain strong. I know you can do it." (I know he can too).

I get caught up in details of the time but always know that I pray for Mike, I must. I talk to him about his friends and family and kids, what I demand he fight for.

My time is almost up, I know he is tired, but as I am getting ready to go, Mike is trying to tell me something... I am leaning in as close as I can to hear him and read his lips...

I just can't figure it out and he is so frustrated. I said OK, I will figure this out I'm not leaving until I understand you. He points at my phone. I hit my homepage. He points to messages. I open that up and to no one he is trying to write a message. The first word is "I," but then he can't get farther... not enough control, letters are too small. Frustration! I say ok Mike, hold on. I get the newspaper I just brought, close the iPad so I could make it a clipboard, and find a pen. Write what you want. He writes "I." I say, the first word, is "I?" He nods. He writes a second word I am trying to figure it out then he does two more words. It's like playing Pictionary. I'm looking and sounding it out and the fourth word is chips. Weird! Then I realize the third word is ice. "I want ice chips."

I'm like you couldn't have written I love you?! He just rolled his eyes. When I left after love taps, Mike was closing his eyes and nurse Esther was hurrying off for the chips. He deserves a few. See you tomorrow my Mikey. Rest up, I have all the belief in the world for your success tomorrow.

Individual Prayer Requests.

Continued strength and healing towards coming home.

Strength of mind and body and confidence to stand tomorrow.

Pray for all these patients, there are so many heart-wrenching stories here.

Prayers for these workers. May they see their worth through the compliments of our community.

Quotes:

Steady As We Go.

"Go, as long as you can, and then take another step (or sit and stand for now)"

"One day you will tell your story of how you've overcome what you're going through now. It will become part of someone else's survival guide."

for Mikey. "If you can't fly then run, if you can't run then walk, if you can't walk then crawl, but whatever you do, you have to keep moving forward."

As always:

Let go and Let God.

Beat the bumps Mikey.

If you ain't cheatin you ain't tryin!

Steady as we go.

Love Sarah

Scripture: Psalm 94:18 "When I felt my feet slipping you came with your love and kept me steady."

Reflection: "How to Maintain a Steady Heart During Trouble."

1) Seek Joy in Christ-even in horrible circumstances.

2) Submit your spirit to God -ask God for control-he is your pilot.

3) See that God is near-he is everywhere. He is **IN** your situation.

4) Send anxiety packing-although things will cause you concern, anxiety is concern out of control.

5) Speak to God about everything-no struggle is too big or small for him to handle.

6) Soak up Peace-your mind can rest, and your heart will be calm.

7) Stay on Top of Your Thoughts-repeat all these steps. -Author Unknown

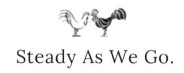

Steady As We Go.

THERE IS NO ME, WITHOUT YOU.

Day 41 / May 18th

I am so proud of Mike. I have loved him for a long time. I guess after time you kind of get comfortable with that love… dare I say we take it for granted. Life gets routine. You talk about your kids, your job, what town you must drive to at night for sports (in a world where those existed).

Mike has always been big in coming home from his factory job and always kissing me, usually on the cheek (did I turn away… and if I did I will never again) and asking about my day. He always cares about how everyone else is. But now I think how often, did I ask him back, "How was your day?" I am sure often, but now I wish more. We would sit if time permitted and have a drink together, discuss the day, who wanted to go what direction that night. Talk about Mike's work buddies and what was happening at the factory (he has an outside job besides the farm), he would ask what houses I cleaned and how it went. Idle chit chat and I hope I never take it for granted ever again. I hope that none of you do either. If you have a chance for a morning kiss or an after-work one, take it. It is so true, don't go to bed angry. I am not saying that I ever did, but if I have learned anything tomorrow is a gift, not to be taken for granted. One day life is good, the next you are spinning. Be happy! Love your one!

Big day today... so here is what I learned about my Mikey, your Mike, your Chicken today. My 5:30 am call to nurse Tara was that Mike had a restless night, he said he just couldn't sleep and during this time he managed to pull his feeding tube out. Otherwise, he was fine, but he is tired. Thank you, Tara... the anticipation of today must have him all riled up. Nurse Marie is the day nurse today. She has not had Mike before, but his reputation precedes him, and she is aware of his ice chip demands. The feeding tube has gone back in. He is doing fine. See you at 2 today. Today I had a friend drive me. Chal drove and her son Seth along with our daughters Alexis and Holly. My girls want to see Mike's new window. They also rent the bikes outside the hospital for a bike ride to the nearest Starbucks they have Google-mapped. They need to have some fun and normal in their world. A little prayer on Mike's outside wall with a double chocolate Frappuccino as a reward.

When I got to outside ICU, Chaplin Claire was just coming out so I took a few moments to talk with her, and may I say, the people she sees in this hospital, if you are of faith or not, she has something to say to you. She is a blessing to this building. I got into Mike's room just as physio did. Mike is in bed, and I go to him... are you nervous, head nod. Mike you are going to do this... I have no doubt, you will do this, you are strong, amazing, you have this. I love you... you do this. Physio is amazing, these girls, (I am sure boys too, but I have not met) can I salute this new department. this department I have been begging to get to meet! I am in awe again. So, Mike sat on the side of his bed, his physio is not easy on him, they do not move his limbs for him... Mike move your leg, Mike move your arm, Mike roll. Sitting on the side of his bed, they bring to him, I will call it a dolly for less technical terms. Feet on the bottom, hands grip a bar and

Steady As We Go.

with physio pull up... he did it! "Mike, chest out, chin up, butt tight. " HE DID IT! Back on the bed... Mike I am so proud, you did it, you did it! I just want to wrap him up. Physio, nurses, all so excited. Do you want to do it again? Head shake no... darn cause you are doing it again and he did it two more times with hard work and such determination and applause ...Gah I love him!   The staff in that room today was amazing... nurse Esther, Marie, and Maddie, you are the tops. Physio. you do cross-fit for a reason. You all have the jobs you have because you are gifted. After 2 hours of hi-flow oxygen this morning (more work for Mikey), 3 stands, an hour in the chair, he got back into bed.

I feel I am getting long again but a few more things. I want you to know Mike loves this staff. They know he loves ice chips, they work to understand him, he smiles at them, he asks for fist pumps, and he thumbs up them. He knows he is doing well but at the same time I leave, and I get a wave, I know he wants to come with. I want to stay. I just pray that all these patients on this unit have the most positive of thoughts, may they believe in themselves and their strength. When Mike stood. One nurse said, "Mike, you let us celebrate you... this is amazing, and we will celebrate." It should be.

I am aware... Mike is a miracle. He is a miracle through the power of prayer, through these people who answered their calling and are doctors and nurses. He is also a miracle through his own determination. There is no quit in him. There is no quit in us... until Mike is home. I know I could talk forever about Mike, so much more I could say but I see his humor, I see his little smile, I see his sadness, I see his frustrations, I see his anger (when he was in his chair), I gave him one of his stress balls to squeeze to work on strength. I backed up and then the ball hit me in the chest.. ok Mike I guess your aim is not so bad after all... frustration wrapped in love. This is a steppingstone... a temporary situation. This temporary leads to the next part of our lives. Finally, because we all know ECMO man I saw him when I was leaving. ...I waved and said "Hi ECMO man." He waved back and came to speak. How is Mike doing? I told him and his eyes lit up even more than they usually do. So proud so amazed and grateful.

Sleep well tonight my Mikey, you deserve it.

Individual prayers:

Prayers for complete healing of his lungs and body to return home.

Strength of mind and confidence.

Secondary infections be kept at bay.

Pray for all these people on this floor, it is a silent floor. Pray for their caregivers.

Quotes:

"The strongest people are not those who show strength in front of us, but to those who win battles, we know nothing about."

"Use your struggles and frustrations today, to motivate you, rather than annoy you. You are in control of the way you look at life."

"Be Mindful."

"I think a hero is an ordinary individual who finds strength to persevere and endure in spite of overwhelming obstacles."

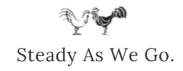

Steady As We Go.

"Don't watch the clock: do what it does. Keep going."

As always,

Beat the bumps.

Let go and let God.

If you ain't cheatin you ain't tryin!

Steady as we go.

Love, Sarah

Quote, *"Without Christ, we might live for the moment, but with Him, we live forever."*

Scripture: "For it is God who works in you, both to will and to work for his good pleasure." Philippians 2:13

Reflection: We are nothing without the loves of our lives- our spouses, our children, our extended family, our friends, our community, and our Almighty Father.

Author Sarah VanNetten

MIRACLE

Day 42 / May 19th

In a world that has gone 'screwy', I am still amazed at the good things you can find if you choose to look. At moments with the state of the world, the sadness, I wonder, is this it? Everything is in chaos, the world is a mess, there is this pandemic that is ripping us apart. To get to the hospital I pass countless shelters and homeless people. To be honest, yesterday when my girls came with me, they were all concerned about what to wear... I am like honestly if you have 2 matching shoes consider yourself blessed. If you have dollars in your pocket for your Starbucks, consider yourself blessed. Put on a shirt and shorts and get your head geared towards what you are doing and let's go. It is unsettling to see the sadness, the sickness, the poor mental health, the tent villages that are occurring right now... I think there are so many opportunities for us to do so many good things... maybe that is what God is trying to accomplish through Mike. I do not believe that God is done with us... no minister I have listened to ever makes mention of that. They look to the future. I think God is teaching us (I have no idea what yet either, but I believe there is good in everything). I know I have seen the good in people's kindness... people are being kind to other people because of Mike, people have beautiful stories to share because of Mike or because of situations they have endured. How many people have been vaccinated because of Mike? How many people have thought, this could be me, or your sibling or best friend? How many have used Mike as a wake-up call? I remember last March taking this lockdown seriously and doing the rules but saying, I know this is serious, but we don't know anyone this has affected...

Steady As We Go.

well guess what. It affected my most important person. I am not wanting to be such a nagger. I just want you to know I don't want this to be you... may I be the only one who you know whoever walks in these shoes and that there is a whole lot of good still left in the world... look for it... Mike is one of these things.

So here is what I learned today about my Mikey, your Mike, your Chicken today. Joanne was Mike's night nurse last night and he did more hi flow oxygen last night. This morning he had a decent night. Sarah is his nurse again today and I will go at 2.

When I arrived today Mike was just finishing up four more hours of hi-flow! Physio had not yet arrived, so I am talking to Mike and Dr. Craig arrives. My gosh, he is so happy to see the improvements after a well-deserved time off that Dr. Craig had. Mike wants to tell him something, but I can't figure it out, so I get the whiteboard. He writes, we cannot read, he is frustrated, but we say go again. One word at a time. He writes, and Dr. Craig reads, "Today is my last day here." I read, then I said where are you going? He mouths "Home." Break my heart, Mikey. Dr. Craig looks at him and says I believe you are, and quicker than what any of us suspected, but we have work to do first so let's do the work. Mike nods his head yes.

Physio girls arrive Ang and Megan. I love their spunk. They get Mike to smile and to work hard. Really who wouldn't want to impress two young pretty girls. Mike does some exercises on the side of the bed for balance and strength, and it is coming. He then does his work using the aid I described as a dolly, but it is called a Sara-Steady (steady as we go). Mike stands three times, but stronger today than yesterday the girls agree. You can see the physical labor this is but fist pumps all around. They move him from Sara, steady to the chair where he spends an hour. It is not his favorite hour to say it mildly. Lots of ice chips and encouragement to get him through it.

We face timed our kids for the first time. It was good for both sides. Short and sweet and will repeat. FINALLY (capital letters needed in Mike's opinion) when physio returns, Mike taps his wrist, looks at the wall clock and rolls his eyes at them. In his opinion, they are late. She gives it back to him and helps to get him back to bed. She told him to rest up, tomorrow is another big day. He will work and use another new support that will require his feet to move up and down and hopefully in a few days he will have a few steps.

Before my good physio friend left, she made the mistake of telling Mike she was indifferent to the Leafs. He turned his head from her and shook his head. I know Mike will still work for the team tomorrow.

Last thing two radio stations shouted out to us today so AMAZING!! Thank you 107.3 out of Tillsonburg (Tilly Town as we like to call it). Thank you to "Country 104" and "Weaver." To hear you know of us is awesome. I also urge you to look at an article shared on my page called "Strides for Health Care Heroes," from Hamilton Health Sciences. I will be sharing this lots over the next little while...For now... I think that is enough. Mike was tired, I hope he can watch some hockey, but rest for tomorrow's Leaf game. I gave him love taps and all our love.

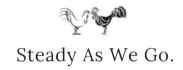

Steady As We Go.

See you tomorrow, Mikey.

Individual prayer requests:

For complete healing for Mike, restored to whole health.

Keep secondary infections away.

For the health care workers and all who have a job within this building.

May we all be vaccinated and a cure from Covid so that we can all get together again.

Quotes:

"Japanese proverb…Fall seven times. Stand up 8."

"Your mind will quit 1000 times before your body will. Feel the fear and do it anyways!"

"No matter how hard it is, just keep going because you only fail when you give up."

"With the new day comes new strength and new thoughts."

As always.

Beat the bumps Mikey.

Let go and let God.

If you ain't cheatin you ain't tryin!

Steady as we go.

Love, Sarah

Scripture: Acts 4:30, "While you stretch out your hand to heal, and signs and wonders are performed through the name of your holy servant Jesus."

"Don't be afraid...just believe." Mark 5:36

"Faith without works is dead." James 3:26

Reflection: We witnessed a miracle. It unfolded right before our eyes. How? We acted. We prayed. The word of God was planted in our hearts. WE waited with patience and with faith. WE expected the impossible. Most of all-WE BELIEVED

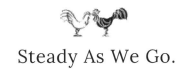

Steady As We Go.

WE ALL HAVE MOUNTAINS

Day 43 / May 21ˢᵗ

Today I find an emotional day. Who does Mike love? The Leafs. and the Jays but a special part of his life is loving the Leafs. It obviously is a part of lots of friend betting and rivalry, but Mike is a die-hard Leafs fan.

This is his night. So, I honestly struggle to be here at home with Mike there. Gah! He should be home on our couch watching his team, but he can't be, and my prayer is that he be home before they win the cup (sorry all non-Leafs fans). I have an iPad there for Mike, but unfortunately, I cannot take my tech crew with me to the hospital. So, I have had to bring it home a couple times…learning, learning, learning. Tonight, although I called down early, I called at, 7: 30. ICU west. A man's voice answered me which does not happen very often. My usual, I am Sarah VanNetten my husband Mike is in this bed number… I know I am early calling, and this will sound so stupid, but I am calling to be sure the Leafs game is on. He answers… "That is not a stupid question at all. That is important. I will go down right now and make sure it is. I may even watch it with him. and if any problems I will call you."

(Can I say that a man answered this phone tonight for a reason) … Now to get onto the injury of John Tavares… (how did I get to analyzing a Leafs game??). What resonates with me is as John left the ice, he gave the thumbs up. let me tell you, thumbs up is hard-core kick-ass strong now. Thumbs up means you have got this. Thumbs up shows that you are strong when others worry for you. Thumbs up shows you are back in the game sooner than you think. Tavares, you are a strong guy, you are now joining the Chicken club... get back, you got this and so does Mike.

So here is what I learned today about my Mikey, your Mike, your Chicken. Mike is spending more and more time on hi flow oxygen which is so good. Extra work! When I arrived at 2 today his nurse is Laura, the first time to have Mike but she is wonderful. I know I say this a lot, so know that this is what these people are. Believe me if I thought my husband was receiving less than great care you would hear. I am not candy coating this, making it sound better than it is... this is as is... Mike receives 1 on 1 care. Mike is sleeping when I get there. Laura shaved his beard today too... He looks so different (I prefer beard but give it a couple days). They needed to see his skin to get rid of some dyes he has received.

Physio arrives promptly at 2. It's gotta be tough to come out of sleep and asked to perform right away... but he did! He did some bedside for his central strength. This is important for balance. Then he stood using a different apparatus today. It had no knee or feet support. On the third time, he lifted his feet too...first steps to real steps. They are so happy with Mike's efforts; he really is doing great. Physio girls put him in his chair for one hour... he checks the clock. 2:30 when he sits. He is getting better at it. The first 45 minutes (SCORE!!) The Leafs as I write, are bearable, the last 15 minutes are work (for both of us). While in his chair the first doctor he had at General stops by. She says, you won't remember me, but I had to come and see you, I saw you when you came to get ECMO, I was there. I saw you in your sickest. I am out of ICU for 3 weeks. I didn't expect to see you when I came back!

Steady As We Go.

Long post ... I long for a short one but ... Mikey did great today. I know he is tired of this. I would call this more of a sad day, but Mike is entitled to it.... this work tires him so much. We had a talk about many things... my gosh, Mike doesn't want this attention, he doesn't want to be cared for, he does not want to be there. Picture yourself as someone needing complete care. He lights up the ICU, he does, but he also now knows where he is. I absolutely love him for it.

Mike and I had a talk about all the people that he has believed in over the years... the kids he has taught to skate, the ballplayers he has taught how to plan. But most importantly the kids who didn't get ice or diamond time and you took the time to take them aside and make them feel like the most important kid on the team. You always do. So now BELIEVE in yourself as you believe in everyone. It is your turn to believe in yourself as much as we do. I told him tomorrow when I come back, I expect his smiles, his fist pumps his little jokes. He is leapfrogging!! Mikey hop on our steady as we go train! I love you so much. Love taps and nap my friend. Watch your Leafs tonight. You will be home soon.

Individual prayer requests

For complete healing of Covid for Mike... Help his lungs continue to improve, may he get off the trach, may he move to oxygen and then his own lungs.

I pray for the mental health of all these patients, patients, and these workers, they are enduring their patient's lives, and stories. May they have the energy for their own families.

Secondary infection is kept at bay.

Quotes: *for tonight the difference between the impossible and the possible lies in a person's determination. Stop waiting for Friday, for summer, for someone to fall in love with you, for life. Happiness is achieved when you stop waiting for it and make the most of the moment you are in now.*

Now every time I witness a strong person. I want to know: What darkness did you conquer in your story? Mountains do not rise without earthquakes.

Love, Sarah

Scripture: "If you have faith as small as a mustard seed, you can say to this mountain, 'Move from here to there,' and it will move. Nothing will be impossible for you." -**Matthew 17:20**

Reflection: Everyone will come to the foot of a mountain at some point in their lives. God knows that He has given you the strength that you need to move or climb those mountains. All we must do is put our faith in Him. Or in other words give him our burdens. He is bigger that the mountains in our lives. Just remember one step at a time, one breath and you will get there. He didn't promise to make it easy, He just promised if we have faith in Him it will move.

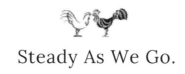

Steady As We Go.

DON'T GAMBLE WITH YOUR FAITH!

Day 44/ May 22nd

Another Friday... a Friday of a long weekend. My gosh how has this much time passed. A hot Friday, that deserves shorts and a t-shirt. A couple of days ago when going to the hospital with my ride Adam, I said to him, "I am wearing jeans because I don't want Mike to know how much time has passed." He looked at me and said, "Sarah, he can look out his window and see the leaves on the trees, the change in the hours of light, he is not stupid, he knows time is passing." Truly, I know he does. I am not sure exactly if he is aware totally. I don't think he remembers being dropped at Norfolk General. When this is all done, I am so curious what's last clear memory is. I know (because I do know) that he heard me all those days, and I know that he felt the power of prayer.

Life lesson tonight. humility. Humility is not a weakness it is a strength. Many people think that humility is a weakness. Mike is learning to walk again. this only makes him stronger. Humility does not diminish our strength and our abilities, but it allows us to be reined in, to be focused. Humility shows growth and confidence. One of the verses that I have read is. "To walk humbly with our God." *Micah 6:8. Is there a more appropriate verse for someone who is learning to walk again with humility.*

Another important day for Mikey… a bit of a pity party yesterday for both Mike and I but tomorrow (now today) would be a new day.

Here is what I learned today about my Mikey, your Mike, your Chicken. Mike is struggling to sleep at night which sucks. They are working hard to figure out how to get him a good night sleep adjusting his sleeping pills and medication. He will get there. It's a learning curve. My visit is at 2 today.

Sam is Mike's Day nurse today and when I arrive, I am gowning up and talking to Sam about Mike and I am partially hidden behind his curtain and after a couple minutes of talking to Sam, I feel a hand exercise ball hit me in the chest. Oh, hi Mike. So sorry to ignore you. Glad your aim is fantastic AGAIN and still. How are you?

He looks good today, a one-day beard growth, his hair is cleaned up. He is doing ok. I tell him how much we love him. This is the care here. Troy part of the ICU team who does not have Mike but has popped into see him comes in and says that he is trying to fast forward the communication department because he wants Mike to be able to communicate as best as he can, so they will be bringing in some "props" to aid him. He gets so frustrated when I don't understand, the eye roll that I missed. Make no mistake they still roll perfectly. I said to him, Mike this is not you, it is me, I am just learning to lip read but you are doing so wonderful. Here, use your white board, write slow, stop after each word so I know a new word is coming. Two hours of charades. But we are both getting better. Physio comes in.

Angela, who Mike has a love hate relationship with. She pushes him. Mike knows that our good friend Gary drove me today (nickname Zooey). Before physio starts, he is

Steady As We Go.

whispering, can't get it, out comes the board. "See zoo." Me, in my head, "You want to go to the zoo, what the heck, then, "you want to see Gary. You want to see Zooey?" His head nods yes. He wants his nurse to take him outside to see Gary. Oh, my Mikey. Soon enough but now you must work. Today we had a few extra specials to me in watching Mike. Believe in yourself Mike, you have this, believe in what we all see in you. First stand, amazing, this is what he did... as he is standing, he holds upright hand supports, he lets go of them for a second and looks at his girls... Mike you are amazing but don't ever do that to physio again without warning them first... you almost heart-attacked us... but secretly they are ecstatic. Stand two, hold it for thirty seconds Mike. Can I tell you about the recovery between these stands...? It is like he ran a marathon, the recovery, the look of pure work. All on hi flow oxygen might I add. Lift three, hold, hold, hold, now lift left, lift right, five times each. AMAZING. Now we are headed to the dreaded chair. But instead of being lifted in, Angela and team make him walk to the chair. He did not get the whole way, but he made it halfway. Angela is kind of like me. She says to Mike, "Mike yesterday I told you, you did a step, but it kinda sucked. I told you that to make you feel better, but today you stepped, you walked, you were amazing, and you know what I wish the Leafs luck tomorrow night. you rocked today."

Thank you, Angela, thank you for believing in Mike, for your tough love. Ok. an hour in the chair ahead of us. I wanted to say that I have said how I am unsure if Mike knows the date. Today is the first day I can remember that on the white board on the wall it says the date... May 21, 2021. Today we Face-Time Woody. I have had an army behind me, make no doubt, I cannot shout out everyone who has supported me, but I have always said to Mike in my bedside talks when he was asleep that I cannot be what he is to his friends, and I cannot be "Chicken" to Woody. For those who know us you know what I mean. The 3 am phone calls, the texts, the love. I am trying my best, but Mikey I can't be the Chicken to the people who need their Chicken. Woody, Mike, and I had a great FaceTime. Mike looked happy doing it. It just left us with those dreaded last 15 minutes. We made it. It tends to be leg massage time. His, not mine, then Angela returns. This is what she says to him. "I know Mike you have big ambitions to get home but the reason I push you, is because until you can spend two hours in the chair, you cannot go to rehab, therefore I push." Mike is back in bed comfortable. Angela tells him she is off till Tuesday, he smiles. Don't worry physio will be on Saturday and Sunday and Monday. Sarah knows exercises for you to do. He mouths thank you, and Angela says you are so welcome. I give Mike one more motivational speech about all our pride and love for him. I set him up watching last night's hockey game, not the Leafs, I don't want him to have to endure that again tonight. They would rather him not nap; they want him to sleep tonight.

One last thing, when I got home tonight, Mike's dad was in the barn, I went out to check on him and he said, "Sarah, I just got a text from Mike." I left him his phone tonight, he wanted it, I took off his passcode and he texted his dad! Then he texted a few more (if you did not receive one. Do not worry he has 1850 texts to go through.). Let him rest. Don't blow up his phone, he needs to rest, he has many emotions right now. He knows who has texted him. in due time.

Individual Prayer requests:

Steady As We Go.

For complete healing and for Mike to be returned home.

For secondary infections to be kept at bay.

That this staff can celebrate their baby steps and may many more patients show them.

That the world be returned to normal.

Quotes:

"Go the extra mile, it is never crowded."

"Be patient. Sometimes you must go through the worst to get to the best. Give time some time."

"Take a deep breath, no matter how hard things seem right now, you can, and will get through this."

"When I wanted to give up, God told me to get up.

As always,

Beat the bumps Mikey.

If you ain't cheatin you ain't tryin!

Let go and let God.

Steady as we go.

Love, Sarah

Scripture: *Hebrews 10:23 "Let us hold unswervingly to the hope we profess, for he who promised is faithful."*

Reflection: God asks us to hold, fold and grow from things that we experience in life. Holding life's cards in your hand. You ask yourself- Which ones do you hold on to-your family, your friends, your faith? The cards that draw you nearer to God-your prayers, scripture, worship music, and sharing your faith with others. Fold those cards that draw you away from the treasured things that you hold dear to you. Let's fold Covid once and for all. Let's fold fear. Let's hold our loved ones close and hold onto and put trust into the one thing that will get us through anything. Jesus Christ.

Hold up your faith card, but also hold it up for all to see. Magnify it, put flashing lights around it and share it. God is so very present at the core of our being.

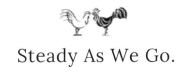

Steady As We Go.

BABY STEPS

Day 45/ May 23rd

I have learned so many skills over these last 45 days. Mostly medical. I have learned firstly what a prone was, I have learned about oxygen levels and what a normal person is as compared to a Covid patient and then a Covid recovery patient. I have learned about the realities of a vent (also know as a breathing tube), then an ECMO machine and what that entails for a patient. I have learned about paralyzing drugs, I have learned dialysis, blood tests, bronch, white blood cell counts. I have learned about circuit changes on ECMO and traches. I have learned about life and death decisions, I have learned how to lean on my faith, to trust God and to say, I give this to you. I give it to you, to the prayers of people and to these people who you have gifted to be so smart that it is awe defying. I have learned way more than I ever wanted to.

At the same time, I have forgotten how to cook, how to make scrambled eggs. I don't care about sorting darks and lights anymore. Laundry is laundry, throw it in and get it done. Different priorities, different realizations of what is important. Different mindsets.

To bring everyone up to date on Mike. He is doing amazing, he really is. I am so proud of him. He is going to kill this part of his recovery. Mike has made amazing strides and will fast track this recovery. Mike was removed from ECMO on May 10th. He is determined, but Mike still has a tracheostomy in his neck, he still cannot speak, he still has not drank water in 45 days except for ice chips. He has not had a meal, only nutrients through his feeding tube, he still receives oxygen through his neck for breath. His bones still feel like they were in a thirty-five-day body cast, his muscle mass is down a lot. Little by little, day by day he will overcome these obstacles.

When he walks, he amazes me, and soon it will be holding my hand... but for now it is with a device that aids him... a walker would be his next step. For now, something a bit more technical. I just want you all to know that Mike is a freaking miracle, he will win before anyone expects but please keep praying.

So here is what I learned today about my Mikey, your Mike, your Chicken today. Night nurse Greg last night. Ok sleep, not great, but he is a farmer, he is not used to a regular sleep schedule, so this is hard for him to adjust. True Greg. Greg is heading on holidays so please enjoy.

Visit today at 2:00. Bernice is his nurse today. So nice to talk to. Mike is doing well. He is doing what he needs. He looks beautiful. Bernice has washed his hair and shaved him looking dapper Mikey. Funny I know it is going to be a one-sided conversation, mixed with charades and hard work, but I can't wait every day to get there. I just want to be with him. I don't see him any differently and I told him, if you think by seeing you sick, I would love you any less you are so wrong. It only makes me love you more. Physio arrives. His favourite. Today my ride, our friends Woody and Chal are standing across the road from his room in an old lot by a billboard.

Today he is to walk to the window. You can do this Mikey. Your goal is to be walking the halls in a few days. You

Steady As We Go.

can do this today. With the help of his physio, he gets up with the aid of his device and he walks to the window. He stands and puts one hand up in a wave. (What drivers see when passing are two crazies jumping and waving and talking to a wall. Welcome to Barton Street). It didn't matter, they didn't care and we were just as amazed. Sit and recover, get stats back under control and stand and use your device to walk your bed length. AMAZING Mike... tiny smile and ice chips. Chair time ... challenge you Mike, you want off this floor, you need more than an hour, let's aim for an hour and five minutes... eye roll. Every time it gets better, a bit better. By the time physio got better it was an hour twenty and it was clear he was not happy... fist in air, point at clock, head shake, but ultimately a smile for them. This is a step. I will share one thing from the chair. Time in the room is always busier between physio, the chair, people stopping; blowing in well wishes. I always pray for Mike while in the room. Sometimes I wonder if this scares him. I have the idea that may have been close to God over this time and had several close encounters to the gates. I don't doubt that his mom and her friends have at several times pushed him back to us...

Today while sitting there, he is folding his hands in and out... you want to pray? His head nods yes. I eye-smile and say Mike I was just thinking I had not prayed today. For us, travel mercies? For workers, for this world, extra love, and prayers always for Mike, but so many people need it.

To sum up I see increased strength everyday, I see his determination, I know his love. I know he wants home, and it is my goal to get him here. I am so proud of Mike. There will never be words to describe my love, nor words to tell of the prayers and thoughts of all of you.

I left him with love taps and watching a hockey game and waiting for a big game tonight... which just happened.

Individual prayer requests:

Pray for Mike's complete healing.

Pray for his and other patients' loneliness and mental health.

Pray for all workers within this hospital.

Pray for Kristin Turner, and her partner Brad in Kansas City. Brad is on ECMO with Covid. I pray Brad follows the same steps as Mike, may he too, be granted healing.

Quotes:

"You'll have good days, bad days, overwhelming days, too tired days, I'm awesome days, I can't go on days. And every day you'; still show up."

"God uses our trials to build our faith. Draw us closer to him and gave us a testimony of his faithfulness for other to see."

"You are where God wants you to be at this very moment. Every experience is part of his divine plan."

As always:

Beat the bumps Mikey.

Let go and Let God.

Steady as we go.

Love, Sarah

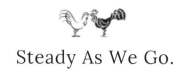

Steady As We Go.

Scripture:

Psalm 119:133 "Allow God to order your steps."

Reflection: God will usher you into his presence as he fulfills his plans, designed specifically for you. It is his will, not ours that we listen to. God knows the day Mike is coming home-he has specific steps laid out for him and is guiding him through his recovery. Every baby step-is a step forward. Forward moving to Mike coming home and baby steps for others towards seeking their own relationship with the holy spirit.

Author Sarah VanNetten

PROUD OF MIKE

Day 46/ May 23rd

Today is a new day... and we have had some good days lately. Mike continues to amaze me. As much as I wish Mike were home here, life continues, and Mike and Kevin's farm continues. Field work is done, grateful to their dad for loving a tractor life. I love all my kids, each special for their own skills and ambitions and strengths but I just want to say that as we approach a new crop of chickens... Mike and I (and all would agree) have only one kid who is a farmer.

Today the barn was readied for chickens with Ryan as our lead. He knew exactly what he was doing, with a little guidance. I have told Mike many times that this farm, these chickens, they are his dream, not mine, do not leave me with them. Don't make me a farmer. You come back to us to farm with your brother, your dad and maybe you can soon take some lessons from Ryan.

My other kids each have their loves. Zack's love is anything but the farm (Brock in the fall and is an amazing umpire and ref). Alexis has an energy that I dare defy anyone to argue with, what she wants she will get and Holly, a little bit of everything, determined, lover, young and a look to the future.

Pamela was Mike's night nurse last night and for the first time, he had a good sleep. That is excellent. I will go again today at 2. Mike, we, our family have received so many generous gifts during this time. None that I can ever repay, but before I left today, our friends, Bob and Sue came by with a delivery. Bob knows someone making a documentary about

Steady As We Go.

the Leafs. He has complete access too. They gave Mike a Leafs jersey signed by the entire Leafs team of this year. Tavares included. Oh my, be still my heart... do you know how thrilled he will be. Over the moon. Thank you, Thank you.

So much to say today so here is what I learned about my Mikey, your Mike, your Chicken today. On my way down today for my 2pm visit, at 1:38 I get a text from Mike which says, "hurry please," are you ok, I am five minutes away... he responds, "I am hot." Mikey you have a nurse. Tell them you are hot and they will give you a cloth, I am on my way...

I also said to him that I know he moved rooms last night like a super trooper and is now a bit farther down the hallway, but I must find you.

When I arrive, Mike is overwhelmed by the jersey, he wants everyone in the room to see it and believe me, he has visitors. People just want to see him and say how proud they are. But Mike is also so anxious, sweating, looking worried... he is going outside. Mike... you can do this; YOU CAN DO THIS. Alida is going to help him..."Mike if I did not believe in you, I would not do this. I do not set you up to fail but to succeed."

The nurse today is Brendan. He is awesome. Room is full of people knowing what this means.

Physio is here. Gosh, weekend girls, weekday girls. How are you so strong? Today Mike you will stand, use your device, and walk out your room, turn, walk thirty more metres out of the ICU into the hallway. The hall you have spoken of. I know you all know he did do it, with pure determination and admiration from these people. Into his chair. He is emotional and winded. (Winded is an understatement). (He is completely out of breath). We are headed outside to the cheers with Alida and Brendan and me. Outside waiting is Woody and Chal. Nothing really can describe I am sure what it was to be outside after forty-six-days and to see people you love, to watch traffic, to see Barton Street. Which can entertain for hours.

Mike does not hear well right now due to his ear infection. Not really a complaint, but he has made it clear.

We spoke loudly, we had friends, caregivers, (who are now friends) engaging in conversation and all centered around Mike. The sun was out, a nice breeze.

Thank you, God. After half hour time to head back. Back we go and Mike we are so proud of you. He is tired. We pass doctors who dealt with him in the early days, eye smile, eye smile. Back in his room where normally a lift back into bed, physio came back in and asked him to stand again and pivot back into bed and although there were several eye rolls and fist shakes, he did it. Back in bed, I leave you with this because I could share the little details forever. As this group of special people (Cousin Chris and Alida. I cannot leave you out of this) gather around Mike's bed, he touches his heart and moves his hands out to them all. I can't ever repay my gratitude, my love. All I can say is that you believed in your ability to heal, your love. Not sure how you do what you do day in and day out, but then I guess it is for a person like this... a miracle. There isn't much that can replace this. When I left, I prayed, I gave love taps and Mike was closing his eyes. He crossed another X off the list.

Steady As We Go.

Individual Prayer Requests

Continue in Mike's healing for complete body healing.

May Mike and all patients on this floor have good mental health... may all people have this; this is not an easy time for anyone.

Continued healing towards being off the trach.

Quotes:

"Take Control of how you feel in every circumstance,

Work on yourself daily,

Your story is far from done."

"The best is yet to come."

"Faith is confidence in God before you see God emerging."

"The journey of a thousand miles begins with a single step."

"The power of determination will make you unstoppable."

"Seeing is never believing, we interpret what we see in light of the way we believe."

As always

Beat the bumps Mikey.

Let go and let God.

If you ain't cheatin you ain't tryin.

Steady as we go.

Love, Sarah

Scripture: Hebrews 11:1, Faith is the substance of things hoped for, the evidence of things not seen.

Reflection:

The overwhelming pain, the uncertainness and shaking of our daily lives can be upon us in a moment. Just as quickly as tragedy can enter, so too is a heart filled overflowing joy. The kind of joy that can come only from answered prayers in faith rewarded, miracles and love that has no limit. God is the source of love and joy; He is the maker of miracles!

Steady As We Go.

DETOURS

Day47 /May 24th

We-ll, the first long weekend of the summer is almost past us... another long weekend in lockdown.... hopefully the last we will ever see. Hopefully our world is on the way to mending. Hopefully we can love and share and hug again soon. This is not the way I ever wanted to spend a long weekend but in the same sense it was a great weekend because of all the progress Mike has made. Mike's progress makes me happy; it gives me a bit of breathing room. I see reminders of his personality shining through. I see him making nurses and doctors smile, I see him giving them his thanks for what they are doing. It is good to see some of what we all are missing so badly.

A good friend sent me a devotion this morning and it struck me how true it was. It was about detours. They come in all shapes and sizes-the common thing about them is we do not see them coming. (How true is that). They catch us off guard, leave us scared, confused, heartbroken. We don't know how long the detour will be. They lead to an appreciation of what a smooth highway is like, and how sometimes even along the way to reaching this smooth highway we can see beautiful scenery along the way. It is easy to become discouraged and question God along the way and our faith is tested. The way he leads may not make sense to us, but he has his reasons for every detour. The detours' purpose is to showcase God's glory as he shows his power through the detours. It is hard to be cheerful (darn hard), during a detour, but look for the good moments and say, "I don't understand God completely, but I trust in where he is leading me as we navigate back to the main road."

So here is what I learned about my Mikey, your Mike, your Chicken today. Mike had an ok night... he struggles with sleep but that will happen in time. His day nurse today is Alyson. She has had Mike before when he was way down the hallway and on ECMO. She is so much happier to have him in this room. Mike is in bed. He has on a pair of his shorts today, fresh shave, hair combed, he looks good. Even though physio is off today, Mike did not get an off day. PT Angela will be so proud of these girls today. This morning they had Mike do what they call a 'dangle', where he sits on the bed side and simply practices balance and breathing with a few pushes to check his balance and improve it. He sat there for 15 minutes. His 2 powerhouse nurses then had him stand... without using a standing device, just their own strength and Mike's determination, which was amazing! Onto his afternoon work. First job... brush your teeth... his dentist will be happy to know he is back to some oral hygiene. It is such a treat just to be able to watch him brush his own teeth... what a joy to see his hand moving and controlling the brush. Chair time now and with his walking aid he stood up and pivoted and backed into his chair. Their goal is an hour, I say he has been able to do an hour 20, he can't do less than that today... not backwards, only forwards... eye roll, eye roll.

Today my girls came with driver Jen. I told Mike when they were under the window, I also watched from the window while our favourite police officer friend helped a sleeping homeless man who was sleeping under Mike's window to perhaps a better place to sleep. I can't wait for Mike to be able to stand at his window... he will be entertained for hours.

Steady As We Go.

Mike is so damn cute... he knows so much about his care now; he can help do things. There is a suction that they use in his mouth, like what the dentist uses... he pretty much suctions his own mouth now. He continues to be on high flow and needed less trach suctions today... none while I was there. Besides the street entertainment we FaceTime with good friends Zooey and the Coch. It was just a good visit, and I was able to figure out mostly everything Mikey was trying to tell them... very little frustration. Just some smiles from Mike, thumbs up... hopes for more normal times. 20 minutes to go in the chair. Every day I see it getting a little easier to get through this. Leg massages, some texting with friends, telling him how proud we are of him... how inspirational he is, how much we all love him. He sat an hour and a half in the chair... his record. PT Angela is going to love this! Don't look back, only forwards, we are getting to that 2-hour chair sit. Mike again uses the aid to get up from the chair and back into bed. He doesn't look quite as exhausted as he did yesterday. I am so proud of him... I say it all the time, but it just thrills me to see these little improvements. His pain is mostly under control. I sat with Mike for another little bit... his calves are sore, so I gave them another massage. I prayed for Mike and for all the leaps he is doing and for continued leaps and for peace and confidence and for these workers. I hate leaving Mike, his eyes leak a bit, mine leak a bit but I said I will be back tomorrow, and you keep doing this Mikey and you will be home before anyone anticipated. After all, you will say you had this the whole time.

I thanked the girls and waved again to Mike. He was watching poker on the iPad, readying himself for the big game tonight. See you tomorrow.

As I walk out of the west and into ICU hallway, I run into my favourite. ECMO man! His eyes light up, mine light up. He asks how today was and I tell him all of Mike's accomplishments today. He is delighted and then says, and how are you doing? I tell ECMO man I am doing ok because Mike is doing better. Thank you for what you did. See you again ECMO man have a good break. Eye smile and a wave bye from him. Bless these workers.

Individual Prayer Requests

For complete healing for Mike for a return to home

To keep secondary infections far away

May we all get vaccinated as quickly as possible to return to a normal life again

Pray for patients, young peoples… everyone's mental health

Quotes for Today

"If it doesn't challenge you, it doesn't change you."

"Success in life comes when you simply refuse to give up, with goals so strong that obstacles, failure, and loss only act as motivation."

"HOPE- if you only carry one thing throughout your entire life, let it be hope. Let it be hope that better things are always ahead.

Steady As We Go.

Let it be hope that you can get through even the toughest of times. Let it be hope that you are stronger than any challenge that comes your way. Let it be hope that you are exactly where you are meant to be right now, and that you are on the path to where you are meant to be... because during these times, hope will be the very thing that carries you through."

As always,

beat the bumps Mikey

let go and let God.

If you ain't cheatin you ain't tryin

Steady as we go

Love, Sarah

Scripture:

Romans 5:3-5, Not only so, but we also rejoice in our sufferings because we know that suffering produces perseverance, perseverance, character, and character, hope. And hope does not disappoint us, because God has poured out his love into our hearts by the Holy Spirit whom he has given us.

Reflection:

Detours- None of us can see the future. We have no idea what lays ahead on our own road. We have no idea how many detours we will be taken on or what they will take out of us. I also don't think we know where our strength comes from until we find ourselves in the midst. For me, it was God and faith in knowing he was in charge. It made it no less scary, but it gave the road a 'sense of peace' that I could feel. I pray that you always feel the presence of God on whatever path and detour you are on.

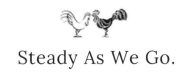

Steady As We Go.

KEEP LOOKING FORWARD

Day 48/ May 25th

So much to be so grateful for. So many things that could have been but didn't. So many walls that we were against but bounced off and out. I remember the first couple days, (which at times seems like yesterday and other times it seems like this has been going on for years), the one thing I remember being told is we are going to have steps forward, we are going to have steps backward we can't get caught up when we take a step back and we must be cautiously optimistic when we get the steps forward. So true... such wise people. Celebrate the uneventful nights, be grateful for the baby steps we saw and be ready to have to get your head wrapped around whatever happens tomorrow. I say this for no other reason than as I sit here writing this with a glass of wine and the Leafs game on... I wish Mike was here. As happy and thrilled as I am with his progress, I miss him. I hate thinking of him watching by himself on his iPad... (although he is never by himself, he always has his nurse and people popping by), he deserves to be home. I am not alone in my thoughts; I know we all want Mike home. I know there are many more husbands or wives who want their partner home and what I am even more aware of is there are many out there who will never have their partner home. My heart breaks for these people because it just doesn't seem fair. Their detour did not lead to the direction any of us would want. It's a heartbreaking, bitch of a virus that baffles and confuses and scares. So as much as I feel sorry for sometimes myself and family and for Mike... I really have nothing to feel sorry for... we are far more blessed than some. Count your blessings friends... count them one by one, keep the pity parties short and the realizations of the blessings huge.

So here is what I learned today about my Mikey, your Mike, your Chicken. When I called down this morn, at 5:30, Mike had a decent night sleep, he had a male nurse. I missed his name, but he was great to talk to, "Oh yah, Mike slept not too badly, he has been up since 4:30, he is just in there on his phone texting away." For those who received a 4:30 am text, count your blessings. I am just so happy his fingers work well enough for him to do this, and it puts some time in for him. The days are long, I am sure. I arrived for my 2-o clock visit. Mike has a male nurse, with the great name of Mike today. When I walk in nurse Mike is up by Mike and my Mike is writing a message to nurse Mike... no idea what they were talking about, but both were right into it. Nurse Mike introduces himself and Mike gives an OK sign and mouths 'Good guy'. Physio girls arrive, they are ready for Mike. Megan and Angela walk in with matching Leafs caps on. They get an immediate thumbs up and slight smile, even though he knows what is coming. Sit on the side of the bed, get your balance, breath, relax, be confident. I get a job today. I am the chair driver to follow Mike on his walk. I told them I am not sure Mike would trust me as I am not even allowed to drive the lawnmower since I tried to help one day and drove the new lawnmower right under a fan in the chicken barn and got it quite stuck. Mike never got mad, he calmly backed the new lawn mower out from the fan with the warped hood now said, "Thanks for the help, but I can cut the grass from now on." Fair enough. Now I have the job of steering this chair in

Steady As We Go.

my opinion, his 'wing man'. I'm sure in his head he is thinking this could go sideways quickly, but he is not calling the shots. Anyway, Mike gets up off his bed with the help of his girls and the aid and then we walk, out of the room and turn a tad down the hall. Got the chair in place and sit and rest, get your breath, stats back to normal. Get up and walk a bit farther. Went as far as he could and sit again.... chair perfectly in place both times. He got wheeled in his chair back to his room for chair sit time. He did well. He sat for at least an hour thirty maybe a bit more. It's not a great time yet, but it is not as painful as it first was (for either of us). Mike gets so hot! It truly is like finishing a workout... spend much time putting cold cloths on his head, leg massages for calf tightness, and repeat. We FaceTime the kids which was great. Told him some of the people I had talked to or had seen, told him our pride, these are huge steps Mike, you are just an inspiration. I prayed for Mike and crew and then we made it through chair time. Leaf girls are back for a stand and a pivot back to bed and a congratulations Mike for your work again today. Mike brightens their day, although he hates it, he knows they are helping him, and he always waves goodbye. He is improving... he knows what's going on and is getting a bit more used to some of these things going on in his body. He knows when he needs his own mouth suctioned and does a fine job at that. He just wants instantaneous... we all do, he wants out, which is great and motivates him. He is doing little things every day to get to that goal. Keep the belief in yourself Mike, keep the faith and know that you have this. There is a cheerleader sitting at the end of your bed, they pop in from the other ends of ICU, they cheer you when you walk. You have cheerleaders everywhere, praying, following, texting you, talking about you. Feel it all and keep moving forward, after all the future is in the forward, you will not find it looking behind in the past.

Individual prayer requests

For complete restoration of health for Mike

To keep secondary infections far away.

Pray for more happiness on this floor. These doctors, nurses, physio, RT, have beautiful eye smiles and they need to be seen more often

Pray for healing of Covid.

Quotes for today

"The best feeling in the world is watching things finally fall into place after watching them fall apart for so long."

"I survived because the fire inside of me burned brighter than the fire around me."

"Falling is part of life. Getting back up is living."

"The pain you feel today will be the strength you feel tomorrow."

As always:

beat the bumps Mikey

let go and let God.

If you ain't cheatin you ain't tryin

Steady as we Go

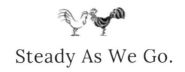

Steady As We Go.

Love Sarah

Scripture:

Proverbs 14:30: A heart at peace gives life to the body, but envy rots the bones.

Reflection:

Count your blessings. When upon life's billows you are tempest tossed, when you are discouraged thinking, all is lost, count your blessings, name them all one by one, Count your blessings, not your troubles.

Never want the things you want make you forget the things you have in your life!

LEAN ON ME

Day 49/ May 26ᵗʰ

Friendship- The definition of friendship is a relationship between people who like each other and enjoy each other's company. An example of friendship is when you have a buddy with whom you like to do things. The definition of true friendship is someone who has your back, no matter what. They watch out for you and ensure you are not in danger. A friend will never purposefully lead you into making decisions that aren't good for you. A true friendship will always have your best interest at heart. There are friends, there is family, and then there are new friends who become family.

I think about Mike a lot, many of us do. This is what keeps coming back to me. This paragraph sums Mike up. Mike is this kind of friend. Mike might as well have his picture beside 'Friendship' in the dictionary. Mike is my best friend... but he is that to others... I know that, and I know he is a great friend to very many more. He can make so many people feel important. because you know what, to him they are. I hate hugging... I have never liked it, don't know why, never my thing. Tough love? I don't even know. But Mike is a hugger, a kisser, a lover, a make you feel more important. I don't think I will need lent again to ever vow to hug more ... I kinda get why people may love it so much, I miss being hugged by Mike. My final point being, I feel that... no, I know that we have new friends who consider us friends and I honesty can say, you have helped to bring us to where we are.

Steady As We Go.

So here is what I learned today about my Mikey, your Mike, and your Chicken today. Although Mike has texting abilities, I still can't help myself, I need to have a nurse's report, so I called down last night and again this morning at 5:30. Mike has Nurse Brendan again... so happy to talk to him again. Mike was happy watching the Leaf game last night, they were making some adjustments to sleep and Brendan this morning said he had a good night. I met Brendan on days this week and I can just picture him standing there with his great upbeat attitude... all these people I want to be friends within another space. Brendan is off for a few days. I hope you get back to Mike. Visit today again at 2 o clock. Mike's day nurse today is Dianne who Mike has discovered went to school with some of Mike's old Friday night church league Jet teammates... how he figures this stuff out is beyond me... I play charades for 2 hours and he has entire conversations with those who surround him. For those wondering why Mike can't talk... he still has a tracheostomy in his neck. It is not removed yet. It is our next goal... to be checked off the bucket list I am sure soon.

Physio girls arrive. Miranda and Michelle today... Miranda tells Mike he may not remember her but was the first person to get him to stand. The physio goal now is for Mike to be weaned from the vent and to be able to use hi flow. It is a gentle balance between the physio and the respiratory therapist. They want him to use hi flow as much as possible... so now it's a give and take. Today not so many bed exercises. Just sat on side of bed for a minute then right up to walk with his device and girls. Nurse Dianne told him she has never dropped one in 30 years so if you think you will be my first get over it, be confident, you will not fall. He went his farthest distance. Prob 90 feet. When he sat in the chair... the applause by all these people who gather in the hall to watch... goosebumps. I can see his steps getting a bit higher... a bit more confident. I can see him able to move his limbs a bit better. Helping him pull himself up from laying. I can see him hating his chair sit but enduring it better... (remember the first day... pound, pound, pound on the mattress, bless his most beautiful heart).

After that walk, that's enough, wheel back to the room, switch back to hi flow. Mike has complained how hot he is... his hair grows so fast and so thick so today I brought clippers and I asked Dianne if she had any experience. She said she would love to, so Mike is now sporting a buzz cut and hopefully that allows Mike to be cooler. These nurses are Jacks of all trades. We go through the rest of the visit with Dianne, texting, talking, praying, anticipating the future. At 4 after hour and a half, physio back and a stand and a pivot into bed. Amazing day Mike. Amazing! He will watch hockey tonight that Jays are postponed. Goodbyes are tough but every, ' See you tomorrow', is closer to home day. Love taps, blown kisses, and I will see you tomorrow.

Individual prayer requests:

Complete healing for Mike that he returns home quickly to us

Secondary infections be kept far away,

Pray for Kristin Turner in Kansas City who is struggling and that Brad's lungs 'pop'

This bastard of a virus is affecting worldwide... pray for immunization by us all, pray for people to see it exists and to

Steady As We Go.

believe and see with open eyes so that this world can be returned... kids can be kids, can we all just see what is happening

Quotes for tonight.

"*On particularly rough days, when you're sure you can't possibly endure anymore, remind yourself that your track record for getting through bad days is 100 %*"

"*Storms make trees take deeper roots.*"

"*You will not be the same after the storms of life, you will be stronger. Wiser and more alive than ever before!*"

"*A rose does not know where her scent reaches, just as a MAN does not know who his life will touch.*"

As always

beat the bumps Mikey

let go and let God.

If you ain't cheatin you ain't tryin

Steady as we go.

Love Sarah

Scripture:

Proverbs 27:9, A sweet friendship refreshes the soul.

Reflection:

Looking back now on these hospital days a month after discharge, it is still amazing to think that Mike is still here with us. I re-read this day's post and it is like I am right back in the moment. I remember writing about the type of friend Mike was to people, trying to paint a picture. Now that he is out, he gets stopped often, some people he knows, others he has never met, but all feel they know Mike and they smile and say how happy they are to see him.

Never take the friendships in your life for granted. Be a friend to those you can see need one. No one should ever be alone in their life without a friend. No one should ever feel that lonely. Be the type of friend to others you wish someone would be to you. Make the world a little bit of a better place through how you are as a friend.

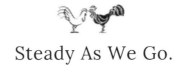

Steady As We Go.

YOU MUST BELIEVE

Day 50/ May 27

My gosh. Where were we all before Covid started. Remember the days kids left the house for school? People left their house for work. They put on pants and makeup. Remember the days we went out for supper, kids went to parties, parents went to weddings or buck and does. Hockey tournaments happened and the beloved hall parties. So many memories that we are all missing out on. I want to have more memories with Mike, with our kids, family, friends. I want to have a normal life. Mike is working his butt off to get back to this. Tomorrow my final 3 kids will receive their first vaccine. Myself and my oldest are done. It is just so important. If they do not have them... they will not see their dad. They want them, they see the future and a return to normal life... but honestly as Mike progresses and eventually comes home, he needs safety, and safety is vaccine... can't keep him safe without it.

So here is what I learned today about my Mikey, your Mike, your Chicken. Mike had a sleepless night, feed tube out again... no fault of anyone but with more movement, it moves and slips. Without a tube, no sleeping help so a long night. He has had sleepless nights before, and he adapts. He is a warrior... but what he really is, as someone pointed out to me is a million little miracles... miracle, after miracle after miracle... keep going and going and going. The fact I can even walk into a room to see him is a miracle. Visit today again at

2. Shay is Mike's nurse today. Young and great. He is doing well... he looks good! His head looks cooler. Speech pathologist Alannah came in, they want to assess his swallowing, want to get Mike onto thickened liquid eventually. She explained everything so well, how the throat works, your vocal cords. Everything about swallowing (another area of expertise that I get to see now). She carries in with her a container of apple sauce and a little thing of some sort of juice. She explains to Mike that she thinks he is ready, she will see how he does and then hopefully book a test to see how his swallowing does. Mike is so excited... he wants this but as she sits him up and gets ready, she says to him... are you ready for this? He mouths, "I just want to do good." Break my heart, Mike you always do good. He did 2 spoons of applesauce and 1 spoon of a thickened lemon drink, and he passed Alannah's test, so tomorrow he is booked to have his swallow checked by X-ray and hopefully a drink is soon in his future... He was so happy. I love to see his smile, to see his eyes crinkle, to see a bit of happiness. He deserves happiness.

Speech leaves and physio arrives. Yeah! We know we want the hi flow used more than vent, so physio came in also in the morn and did exercises in bed. I told him he may leave more fit than he came which earned a giant eye roll. Time to walk. Confidence is the thing. You can, you will go farther than yesterday. Mike this is old news, you know what you are doing. BELIEVE. Come on Mike its time... you have this. Up he gets, straight, tall, head up, butt tight, look forward. Confidence Mike. I was chairperson today again (so proud to have a part). I shout encouragement from behind, not sure he can hear since he is kinda deaf right now in an ear, but I don't care. He makes it in one walk 10 feet further than yesterday. Awesome Mike, you have amazed and made these people's jobs worth it again. When he sits with chair in perfect

Steady As We Go.

position, sweat pours down his face... walk 100 feet. Would your face pour sweat? Would you need a monitor to recover your stats? would you need a vent or hi flow oxygen to do it? A chair ride back to the room and a chair sit now for hour and a half and a few. First half went by fast. Lots of doctors popping in... at times I think I am living Greys Anatomy (and to give these health care workers the respect they deserve... that is how I intend it). We had a doctor today who was a resident of the cardiovascular team, he came in with the most amazing confidence. Told us he was the best there was and I believed him. He came to help with Mike's feeding tube which has given trouble time and time again. He fixed it. When he was done, I said, "Aren't you a heart doctor?" Yes, I am. I said then I bet you are happy you could fix that nose tube with ease! His eyes smiled and said yes it wouldn't have looked good if I didn't. I love these people all helping each other in whatever way they can.

Anyway, long enough tonight. We got through the sit. Stand pivot turn back to bed... (since tonight is the Friends reunion, I can't help to say that every time I hear the word pivot now, which is every day, I hear Ross... PIVOT, PIVOT, PIVOT. I still smile). Mike is settled watching the Jays. You know I prayed; you know all the things I said. I love tapped; I just love him. See you tomorrow my Mikey.

One last thing... Mike has had the same roommate for quite some time. He has struggled but today he received news of improvement. It is not rocket science. These curtains aren't soundproof, they know how Mike is and I know how he is. His dad is always his visitor. Tonight, as I leave, I say to him, I am so happy you had improvements. Thank you. He follows me into the hall and just wants me to know that he understands what COVID has done to Mike... he has gotten his shot and he has told his family about this strapping farmer that is Colton's roommate and that he can personally validate that this is real. Please get your shots. He is so happy they are getting them. We talked for a minute about how each of our lives have changed, in the blink of an eye. We will move together in the same direction. Strangers brought together who otherwise most likely would never have met. Another part of the scenery along this detour towards our paved road.

Individual prayer requests.

Complete healing of Mike's body from Covid

Secondary infections be kept far away

For a good night's sleep

Pray for Colton, for Mike, for Brad, for .... (Put in a name), so many need prayers.

Quotes for tonight:

"Believe in yourself and all that you are, know that there is something inside of you greater than any obstacles."

"The comeback is always stronger than the setback."

"Look up

get up and

don't ever give up!"

"Beautiful irony is when the very thing that tried to destroy you. instead made you stronger."

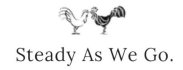

Steady As We Go.

As always:

Beat the bumps Mikey

let go and let God.

If you ain't cheatin you ain't tryin

Steady as we go

Love Sarah

Scripture:

2 Corinthians 5:7, We live by faith, not by sight

Reflection:

Believe: To accept as true… to be sure of the truth

Confidence: The feeling or belief that someone can count on something or someone It is almost like these 2 words are the same… they go together so often. These were such 2 important words throughout Mike's stay. We talked about them so much …. Believe in yourself Mike, have confidence you can do it. Believe in yourself and believe in these workers who so believe in you. In today's times of low self esteem and mental health issues, I think these are two such important words that we can't forget about. Urging positive belief in ourselves and others and to see confidence in people and in ourselves is so important. None of us are perfect enough to cast judgment of others.

Author Sarah VanNetten

Believe in yourself, love yourself and have confidence that you are doing your best!

SARAH AND HER COUSIN CHRIS (ONE OF MIKE'S NURSES)

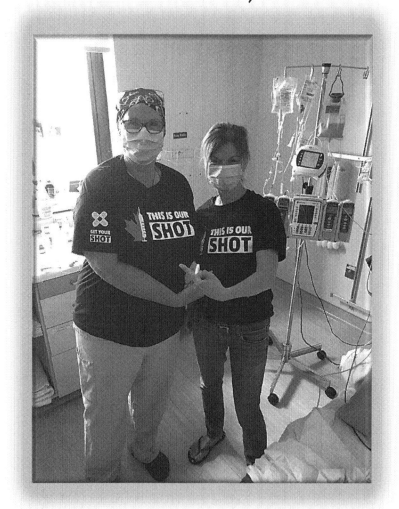

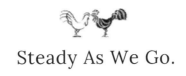
Steady As We Go.

GINGER ALE
Day 51 / May 28th

Going back to day 1- April 8th, it took me forever to scroll back that far but I found it eventually and got there. A post on that day from a scared, frantic, heartbroken wife has turned into something I could never have imagined. The things Mike's body has gone through, the ups, the downs, the good moves, and the devastating talks. There has been a lot in 51 days… so much so that it is hard to believe. Was that really that many days ago? My gosh, he fought back from that position. We have met many wonderful people along the way. I went from 392 likes, 170 comments, 10 shares (pretty much all my friends). I am now at 1300 likes, 300 comments and, about 150 shares on a post. You know what… I love it because it means people are thinking about Mike, they understand, I hope, how real Covid is, they are getting their vaccines and they are appreciating their health care workers in their immediate circles. I never wanted this, but I truly believe that Mike is making a difference across the country. Mike could be your neighbour, your best friend.

So here is what I learned today about my Mikey, your Mike, your Chicken. When Mike texted last night during that not-so-hot hockey game, Mike was tired. They joke up there that Mike's sleeping pill is like a horse tranquilizer. I asked him if he had his horse pill yet, he said not yet but soon. He did not see the third period or OT (phew). When I called nurse Pam this morning, he had a good sleep. Today Mike had his swallow test. I got a sad text from him that he failed. Oh, my Mikey, that's ok, you will get it next time. I am leaving home; I will see you soon. When I arrived, he was sad. I told him first off no one uses the word fail on this floor so never use it again. I told him physio was coming in a few so concentrate on his walk. He just waved at me and mouthed 'Taking day off'. I said, "You're not taking a day off Mike, a day off does not bring you closer to home so when these girls come in you will walk and you will walk farther than you did yesterday. Don't be sad, get mad. Focus on what you can do and walk." Physio arrives, and they see Mike's sad eyes. Angela talks to him, and he is ready to go. Squeeze your butt, Mike. When you tighten your glutes, everything is taller, straighter, your shoulders, your head, legs are stronger. He stood and walked with his device....as I am trying to catch up with his blasted chair that has 1 wheel I can't get to turn; the dietician comes in and says I have a surprise for Mike when he returns. Perfect but I gotta get my wheel turning here and catch up... I can't not succeed on my job. Mike through motivation from every room he passed, made it his farthest again today. YES Mike. It was amazing to watch. My heart pounds every time. Wheeled back to his room, put back on hi flow for the chair sit. Dietician Michelle is waiting, and speech pathologist Alannah is there as well. They explain that Mike did not fail like he thinks, he did ok. I watched the x-ray's of Mike swallowing. He is not quite there on full liquids like water and thick things like puddings, a bit of those go the wrong way into his lungs. He does well on the slightly thickened liquids. Since the first time Mike has met dietician Michelle or Barb, Mike has written them the message, "When can I have ginger

Steady As We Go.

ale?" Mike's special treat was a thickened ginger ale. His eyes and his mouth when he got a spoon of thickened ginger ale was just amazing. They gave him what he has wanted. Even better, if his oxygen level stays good, Mike will be receiving a thickened chocolate milk for breakfast and supper, and a thickened apple juice for lunch... his days can now be broken up by meals! Amazing news and he is so happy. Because he spent time in chair this morn for test and now, his time is shorter, and he is back in bed in a seated position. I want to say his nurse today, another man was so good to Mike. Mike gave me an OK sign several times and would point to muscles and point to nurse Hazma. He is strong. Was so nice to meet him.

Finally, Dr. Craig comes by to check in... Oh, this man, the happiness and joy you can see. Wow, Mike I just am so happy to see how good you look. He can't say I am amazed because I know he believed it the whole time. He is one of the most brilliant people I have ever had the fortune to meet. He is thrilled, I can see it in his eyes. We will forever be grateful. Thank you as well to Alida VanHamme. Your constant checking in and reassurance to Mike is what the doctor ordered for him. I left Mike with the usual love taps, knowing that he is looking forward to chocolate milk for supper and a new day, one day closer to home tomorrow.

Individual prayer requests:

For complete healing and return to old... even better health

For the staff of this floor. For a success story of this pandemic

For those who have lost people to Covid… this just is not fair.

Quotes for tonight:

"People always say that motivation doesn't last. Well, neither does bathing- that's why we recommend it every day."

"My strength did not come from lifting weights. My strength came from lifting myself up when I was knocked down."

"The hard work puts you where the good luck can find you."

"Be somebody who makes everyone feel like a somebody."

As always:

beat the bumps Mikey

Let go and let God.

If you ain't cheatin you ain't tryin

Steady as we Go.

We are all Waiting for you Mike with our first shots. Hurry home.

Love, Sarah

Scripture:

1 Timothy 6: 15-16, Which God will bring about in his own time-God, the blessed and only ruler, the King of kings and Lord of lords, who alone is immortal and who lives in unapproachable light, whom no one else has seen or can see. To him be honour and might forever.

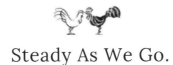

Steady As We Go.

Reflection:

As I read back through my notes, I made on this day on May 28th I see this is what I wrote...Faith has a power because it is confidence in what we hope for and assurance of what we do not see. That is what we put our trust in. God promises that when you draw near to him, he responds by coming closer to us. It is true. As a believer you put your whole trust into something you can't physically see or feel. Sometimes the idea of that baffles me how that can be. If you really wrap your head around putting your hope in something we only know is there because we have seen the evidence of God's work. We can see him in the simplest of things in a day. If we look, he is there. I am so grateful for this gift.

CHA, CHA

Day 52 /May 29th

I will start this today with something that someone told me... A Dr. once told me: 'The best medicine for humans is love. Someone asked, ' What if it doesn't work?' They smiled and said: 'Increase the dose!' How accurate is this? How much does love truly heal and motivate? Love is when you choose to be at your best when the other person is not at their best. Love is when what YOU want is never important. But what the other person needs and wants is always paramount. To truly love is a selfless act. How true are the words when you look up the meaning? But I also know of the love that all kinds of people now have for Mike. They may not know him in the way that some of us do... but they have a vested interest in Mike, and I know through these days of posting they have a glimpse of his life and how could you not love him! Today was Mike's 'person's' birthday... Woody. I know how much Woody loves his birthday, (those of us who know, Woody know how much he loves it). I also know his love of his Chicken so no doubt he would be in the streets of Hamilton today. Not together, but together in a FaceTime from a hospital room to the street below. They are lucky to have this relationship, soon enough back in person but till then, secret handshake and see you soon.

Here is what I learned today about my Mikey, your Mike, your Chicken. Mike had a decent sleep on my early morning call. He was awake and watching some shows and texting. (Early bird catches the worm). Mike had nurse Hamza again today, so glad. Mike loved him yesterday. Looks like a

Steady As We Go.

football player with such a kind and soft voice. He can literally pick Mike up by himself and put him from chair to bed he is so strong. So considerate and attentive. When I arrive, Mike is laying in bed. His eyes are yellow. I am like what is happening, he gestures about not being able to see... Oh no... but then he flashes 10 fingers, 10 fingers and whispers 20-20. Eye test and of course perfect vision. He needed a test due to all the 'stuff' that happened in him, and he passed with flying colours. Physio can't be here till 2:30 so as a bonus Mike you can sit in the chair from 2-2:30. Mike also managed high flow all night and all day today. That's big. Physio today is Elyse and Yvonne. (That is what she is called), so small and a spitfire, but do not mess with either of them, do not be deceived by size. They can manhandle anyone. Big talk about Mike and what he needs to start accomplishing...you must walk farther; you need to be able to be on hi flow as soon as work out is done. We believe in you. Yvonne says, I want you to be successful, I want you to the next floor by next weekend. Ok... Yesterday Mike walked 30 metres, and today they measured, and he did 84!! Talk about success. I don't need to tell you the reaction all around. There is a lot of sadness on this floor, and Mike is providing hope. He is providing hope to the staff, to his family but also to other patients and their families, where there is fight, there is a way back. His work was rewarded with another hour and a half chair sit... and the best green popsicle I think he has ever tasted. We watched some videos, I caught him up on the nothingness that everyone is doing. I prayed. When the time came to go back to bed, Nurse Hazma got called away. To be honest at that moment, he was being pulled in 3 different directions, at the same moment and never once showed stress. I have told you they all have individual nurses (which they do) ... but sometimes more than one is needed for things happening up there. He returned apologized, gave his thanks that things went well in the other room he had been called to and got back to work.

Wise words from a wise friend. How do we get to the place where we walk from faith and not by sight? You must PIVOT. A pivot is a little change in direction, a new path, a new perspective. Sometimes we must trust that God's option is better than what we can dream of, and I believe that Mike is going to come out of this a stronger person than when he went in. I am not sure it is possible to be kinder but that God is full of little surprises.

Mike was resting in bed. We prayed; I love tapped for all. Leaving sucks, it can't not but he is going to do this amazing thing. He will Succeed. I think he finally believes it. I love him with my heart and soul. I am so proud of him; I love looking at him and watching him and even trying to understand what he is saying. It means he is still here, from day 1, post 1, that is all I have ever wanted... the fact that Mike has given hope to people, prayer chains, and people praying who never did pray or believe before, vaccines are increased, covid is real and wow... these people that work in this building are amazing... if you know Mike, you can hear him saying, 'Must be nice.. of course, this would happen.'

Individual prayer requests

For Mike's complete recovery from this most dreaded monster.

For the good mental health for all.

Steady As We Go.

Mike shares a floor with car accident victims, open heart surgery, many other sad stories, pray may they all be healed.

pray for people to believe in God and pray.

Quotes for tonight:

"One day the mountain that is in front of you will be so far behind you, it will barely be visible in the distance. But the person you become is learning to get over it. That will stay with you forever. And that is the point of the mountain."

"Courage doesn't always roar. Sometimes courage is the little voice at the end of the day that says, I'll try again tomorrow. "

"An arrow can only be shot by pulling it backward. When life is dragging you back with difficulties, it means it is going to launch you into something great. So just focus and keep aiming."

"This last one is for physio Yvonne, Yvonne (I heard her say to Mike in the hallway today cha-cha). Optimist: Someone who figures out that taking a step backwards after a step forward is not a disaster, its a cha-cha."

As always,

beat all these bumps Mikey

let go and let God.

If you ain't cheatin you ain't tryin.

steady as we go

Love Sarah.

Scripture:

2 Chronicles 15:7, But as for you, be strong and do not give up, for your work will be rewarded

Reflection:

My families last year have been plagued by poor health .... I am hoping that Mike will be the end of that cycle for a long time to come, but obviously that is never a promised assurance. I used to wonder to myself why for the most part that I had had a smooth life, I had not really been tested. God doesn't give you more than you can handle. To myself I thought, I guess God does not think I can handle much. I compare it to the year at my family Christmas where the many tasks are being divided and the food being assigned, and I got the 'fancy jello'. First off who even eats jello and really? That's what you think I can handle? Well, let me tell you, fancy jello is not so easy. Getting all those layers to firm up on top of themselves and get the fruit floating in the middle, harder than I thought. My point being... at that time I had all I could handle with that jello, and in the same regards God either heard me doubting myself or it was my time because he put a whole lot more on my plate. I have not handled it all with grace, I bumbled, I mis-stepped at times, but I handled it. I'm still here. God knows what he is doing. If he brings to you it, believe in him to get you through it. He knows how much your shoulders can handle.

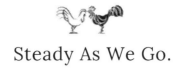

Steady As We Go.

STAY GROUNDED

Day 53/ May 30th

Sunday today, so I listen to different churches on Sundays. I'm requiring a big faith bank these days and I am more than grateful for many messages. What I learned this morning is that we are 15 months into a pandemic (we all know this but when we hear it put into the number of months, it really is astounding). Lives have been changed... we know. People are feeling even more that life is against them, I have felt it myself for about a year now. What people forget is that Jesus is for them. We, as a society need to be more for the people who feel life is against them right now. There are so many, whether it be physical, mental, financial.... people need people right now.... in the ways we are allowed to be. You may be the only kindness someone else experiences today. Sunday is not the only day God works... he works everyday! He takes NO days off, and I guess it is a good thing, that he works everyday because Sunday seems to be Mike's favourite day to need his extra assistance. Most rocky days for Mike have been Sundays ...God's Day, so put him to work. Mike didn't have a great night. He had a fever; his blood pressure was not under control. Possibly some of the popsicle did not end up in the right spot. The thing about this time, is Mike is aware of it, he is awake for this day... he is afraid, he is scared. He has multiple doctors in his room deciding what to do, and although this has happened before, he is now seeing it. Scared doesn't lead to good breathing or blood pressure. This is what is amazing about these people... they figured him out. They figured out the problem, they put him on vent so he could have extra help and they started an IV to get the right medicine into him. I was going to include the following statement in last night but didn't for some reason. I now know why, because God wanted me to save it for tonight... so here it is. "It is hard to stay grounded when everyone including God says you are special. But we must. If we have achieved some success, we must appropriately celebrate the accomplishment and accept the congratulations, but we must keep moving. Come down the mountain, asking God to continue to guard our heart and our steps". (Do not get ahead of God... is how I take this).

So, here is what I learned about my Mikey, your Mike, your Chicken today. I went down early today. Might I say that this morning was the first morning I did not call at 5:30. I thought Mike can text me, I am good. 6:15 I text him and he says, not good... fever. I call as quick as I can dial and am spoken to by the most reassuring people. He is under control, he was scared, we have him on antibiotics... I say to her how this is the first morning I have not called, he can text now, I didn't want to bother. Her response, that is why we are here... for your peace of mind. Please call us... lesson learned.

Mike looks good when I arrive. He has nurse Bill today. Bill is one of a kind. He stays busy the whole time, he is a chatter, he does not like the Leafs, he likes Buffalo, he does like chicken wings, although not until later in life, he makes a mean bed, but he is also a great caregiver. They got Mike back on high flow first thing this morning. Physio will still be coming at 2. Good, we must look forward. I talk to Mike for awhile. I told him that I have put my trust in these people for 53 days, many without you knowing, they have never steered me wrong... you trust them with your might. They have you.

Steady As We Go.

Physio girls are in at 2:00. They realize he had a bad night, but still, we must move forward. We are going to walk but will find a balance between 2 days ago and yesterday. As discouraging as some things are for Mike… if we don't keep our head up, we have nothing. I don't think he felt like walking today, but he wants home, so he walked, and he did it so well. He is so much stronger in getting up. Using his aid, the girls are there but he is doing so much of the work. His respiratory therapist during the walk is so pleased with his numbers. Bill has the IV and I have the chair. What a squad coming down the hallway with Mike as our lead. He does it. I can't even explain my pride. Walks back into his room and into his chair for the sit. Darn he hates it- this chair time. His back and bum which aren't used to sitting, hurt, but everyday does get better. Today we FaceTime his dad and my kids together. It was good. It's ok to show love, but we all must show strength, and that is what took place. Back in bed at 4:15. Took a bit to get stats back to normal… but he did it without going back to vent. Mike is now reading these posts sometimes and I am so proud of him. To hear in Mike's lungs what he is trying to cough up, the work involved and the energy. To see suctions happening through the trach to remove 'junk' from your throat, knowing it is painful, but at the same time a relief. I am getting more used to the struggle, but the suctions get me every time. I say this because once again I never want anyone else to watch this. Mike got settled down, but I stayed a while longer just to be with him. He was watching the Jays game when I left (another disappointment … they struggle with Sundays too I guess).

Ok time to wrap up. A new week in our view... not just for Mike but for everyone, so make the most of it. Be happy, set a goal, do something amazing, pay it forward in some way, say a prayer, be kind, step outside your box, make a friend, do an eye smile to a stranger... be the kind of person the world needs right now.

Individual prayer requests:

I pray for Mike to sleep tonight, for fear and secondary infections to be kept far away and for leaps this week

I pray for these most amazing workers. To listen to them is just awe like

I pray for our world

Quotes for today:

"God is the wind.

Faith is the sail.

You are the vessel.

May you be blessed with smooth sailing."

"I hope you find the time to remind yourself that you are where you need to be, and you will get to where you want to be. (Kinda more for me)"

"In life, the things that go wrong are often the very things that lead to other things going right."

"We will move forward, we will move upward, and yes, we will move onward."

As always:

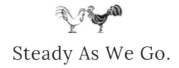

Steady As We Go.

beat these bumps my Mikey

Let go and let God.

If you ain't cheatin you ain't tryin

Steady as we go.

Love Sarah

Scripture:

Isaiah 55:8-9, "For My thoughts are not your thoughts, nor are your ways My ways," says the Lord. "For as the heavens are higher than the earth, so are My ways higher than your ways, and My thoughts than your thoughts."

Reflection:

Staying grounded, achieving successes, accepting the congratulations but then moving on... grounded again and repeat. Reminds me a bit of baby steps. Never getting ahead of yourself in anything really. Never taking anything for granted in life.

Each little success Mike had was a result of amazing medical staff and God. But occasionally, we would get a reminder... like a fever... don't stop praying, don't stop believing, I am still in control. Give the credit where it is due, revel in your accomplishment but then ground yourself again in faith and humility. Asking always for God to be with us. He is not a needy God but an all-knowing God!

Author Sarah VanNetten

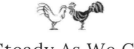

Steady As We Go.

NO DO OVERS

Day 54/ May 31st

I never want a 'do over' in life because I am completely happy with what my life is. I love my husband, 4 great kids who we are so proud of. Kids who do well in school and are athletic and kind. They make us proud. I will say... in all honesty if I could have a do over, it would be in my choice of a career path. I am in admiration of these people. I see more and more everyday all the different career paths even within one building. My mom was a nurse while I was growing up... I was terrified of her job. She worked on the geriatric floor (old people floor), and I remember so clearly back in the days when it was allowed, walking over from the high school to West Haldimand, going up to the 3rd floor to wait for her 7-3 shift to be done and sitting in a wheeled chair in the nurse's station and just spinning it around and around so none of them could 'get' me. ... possibly I was not as athletic as I thought. I also remember when Mike's Beppe was in the hospital and not well. Mike and I were visiting with her with his parents. Beppe was having blood taken and she looked at me and asked... "Are you ok Sarah?" I was not. Suddenly blood work is abandoned, and a chair is under me, and the nurse has forgotten about Beppe for the moment. I have come a long way... we all have. I am, we all are capable of things we never thought possible. It is inside all of us, we must bring it out. Gone is the scared 15-year-old of 90-year-olds in wheelchairs and now is the girl (I hate the word woman) who can walk through an ICU of sick people to get to the bed of my most important. If I could go back... I would be a nurse, or a physio or a doctor. Mike has doctors, nurses, perfusionists, infection team, respiratory therapists, nutrition, speech and language, physio, portable x-ray. I am sure I am even missing someone but all these specialities... we are lucky to live where we are... once again blessed.

So here is what I learned today about my Mikey, your Mike, your Chicken. I called last night before I went to bed and I called back down this morn at 5:30. Good night, on high flow all night. Mike often complains about being hot (sometimes a fever, sometimes not) but one thing I learned today which I did not know was from nurse Lori. The hi flow, or vent oxygen that they put into Mike's trach is warm... the lungs like warm, moist air, so it is not cool air shooting into his throat. It makes him hot... I am sure I had learned this previously, but my brain is holding a lot of things it never really wanted to. When I arrive Mike is sleeping, He looks so darn cute laying there with a cold cloth on his head and just finally sleeping. I sit in his 'chair'. He wakes up shortly as they want to put another iv into his one arm and remove a pic line... we are all about eliminating secondary infection... we just can't chance something being in his body, so get it out. Mike's nurse is excellent. She has a connection to home and Mike writes it out on his phone. I already know this connection. He has had her before, but he would not remember. I tell him yes, I know, she is amazing. Physio in at 2... Angela. Ready for work? Eye roll, head nod. Great. New lesson for today is to use your hands to push off bed rather than using the walker handles to pull. She demonstrates everything (she would rock at charades). I have chair, nurse Lori is on iv pole and Angela has Mike. I know last was in metres but tonight we measured in feet, and he did 195. As

Steady As We Go.

we walk into the hallway, ECMO man is there... ECMO man! He walks with us, as he should, this is his success. His words, "This is just brilliant, beautiful, this is just brilliant!" If his eyes could have smiled any farther. After, Mike sits in the chair to recover... Mike has never really 'met' ECMO man, I say to Mike, "Mike this is ECMO man, I just love him". Mike fist out and a fist pump and a mouth thank you. As always, ECMO man, "No thanks needed, so happy to see you."

Return to room. Good walk, chair time... yeah! Let's be honest, Mike has goals, he wants out of there, he still has concerns obviously, he is still in ICU, so now it is time to set goals. You want out by this date, then let's get the work done, do the walk, work hard, if they think you have more in you... you do. If they think you can sit 10 minutes longer in the chair, you can. You have a goal, lets make it happen because everyone has things they are striving for. Everyone has a goal in their lives. Set one and then focus your eyes and your heart on it. Mike made his chair time. Back to bed and I watched his nurses help him without a walking aid. (I was only in charge of cords and cables for this). I watched the effort in his face to pull his legs into standing, he did it... back in bed and a nice recover. We talked for awhile, I hate to think about going. He knows he is where he needs to be, but it still sucks big balls to leave him.

But I am only leaving for a short time... so that we can have whole days, months, and years soon. Put on hold for some months for years ahead. Mikey knows it too. Believe in yourself, believe in your goals and let's keep baby stepping forward.

Individual prayer requests:

I pray for Mike's complete healing and for secondary infections to be kept away

For Mike and everyone's peace of mind and confidence

I pray for all medical staff, as well as the sanitizers, the cafeteria, the security... all

Quotes for today:

"Success is the sum of small efforts repeated day-in and day-out."

"Be strong. Things will get better. It may be stormy now, but it never rains forever."

Ecclesiastes 7:14. "On a good day enjoy yourself. On a bad day examine your conscience. God arranges for both types of days so that we won't take anything for granted."

"Keep pushing yourself forward. Do whatever it takes. You'll soon leap over the final hurdle and land right where you want to be."

As always:

Beat the bumps Mikey

Let go and let God.

If you ain't cheatin, you ain't tryin.

Steady as we go.

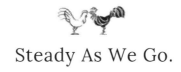

Steady As We Go.

Love Sarah

Scripture: Galatians 6:9, Let us not become weary in doing good, for at the proper time we will reap a harvest if we do not give up.

Job 22:21, Submit to God and be at peace with him; in this way prosperity will come to you.

Reflection:

It's not about being perfect... it's about effort. How true is this! If we had waited for perfection, Mike would still be in the hospital.

How many of us struggle with being perfect though? It generally leads to disappointment because we fall short and then are disappointed in ourselves and feel our efforts were not good enough. I guess that's why it's important to always have effort. There was no perfect cure for Mike in the hospital, he was a learning case, a mass of combined, amazing efforts that moved him forwards. Physio then and now is not about perfect, it's about effort, effort to improve, effort to work towards being the best Mike he can be. Perfection is an ideal we will never achieve, and we will always feel lacking. Happiness will fall short. How much happier will we be to always try and work and be our best and our kindest and we will feel as close to perfect as humanly possible.

THE BIG PLAN

Day 55 /June 1st

Today is the turn of a calendar. June 1. Last month of school, whatever that may look like. I would love for our kids, all of ours to get to see kids in real life, but I understand the pros and cons of both sides to this. I do not want to be a decision maker in this whole thing. You are either loved or hated. Who could possibly know in this world? Trying their best to make the right decisions…we all are.

I know many people who have received their second vaccination… that's amazing! We are getting there. It is what we need. I say this as a person who has witnessed the side affects of Covid. If you have a nice breath tonight, be grateful. I am not saying that Mike and I lived the perfect life. We were careful, but we both worked, we tried our hardest… and if that is you, and you choose not to be vaccinated, then I hope you never see a suction or hear a cough from a Covid patient.

But today is about the bigger picture. I know what I want the bigger picture to be, but it is sometimes hard to see it when you are stuck in the middle. In a predicament because we don't understand that there is a big plan. God has a purpose he needs fulfilling. We are in the middle of this plan. He makes it hard and tough (yes, he does). We want to go around it, but he wants us to go through it- start to finish, to get the big picture. I believe my picture is forming into a clear and nicely cropped view… I believe with my heart. I challenge all those who don't to pray, I know it has power. It can do a heart well, it can heal.

Steady As We Go.

Here is what I learned today about my Mikey, your Mike, your Chicken. Nurse Alannah said that Mike had a good night. Very disappointed in the Leafs, but otherwise, he slept well. I told Alannah to go back and tell Mike, for the first time I think he had the easy end of the night being there instead of at home dealing with Zack and Ryan and the loss from the playoffs of their beloved Leafs. This is what I know about the amazing Toronto Maple Leafs... they are waiting for next year for Mike to be an active participant in the quest for their cup... he quite well has a jersey per night. They are an amazing kind-hearted team that all signed a jersey for Mike. Their generosity with acknowledging the services of front-line workers, by giving them a jersey and tickets for seats that are worth over $2500.00 free of charge. It says a lot...always go blue and white...just saying Habs fans.

Mike had a good night last night; he is on hi flow. (damn popsicles) Today is the day they have decided Mike can go outside again... may I give a shout out to Alida VanHamme who has just worked so hard for Mike. As has my cousin Chris... as has everyone. I arrived at 1 today, Mike is on to walk outside after workout, call home quick, kids on way. Mike looks good. He already has his workout socks on and that's because he has already sat an hour in his chair this morn... He needs to sit for his thickened fluids... fantastic. Miranda arrives at 2 for physio. A few new exercises in bed and then a new walker... a 2 wheeled walker, what we would all picture. With his new walker and trying to sit himself up and pushing off mattress to stand and use this new walker Mike walked 258 feet. He walked 67 feet farther than yesterday with a 2 wheeled walker. Miranda... thank you for pushing him.

Outside with nurse Laurie, RT Alida, and me to see the kids... emotional, yes, therapeutical, no words. The pictures that follow... therefore I believed. At first, I know Mike does not want his picture so I asked the kids to stand in front of the chair and I would get Dad from the back. He shook his head and said no. Mike has not wanted people to see what is happening, but I couldn't be prouder. This is the picture I begged for 55 days ago. This is the proof of YOU Mike. I am so proud, you are beautiful. I want to just show how far you have come to everyone.... therefore, I never gave up... for these pictures. It has been an emotional day. Back to our room for more chair sit. Back to bed, countless check ins. I know we are getting there. I (we) have believed from the start. I do believe Mike is believing now too.

Individual prayer requests:

For complete back to pre health (maybe better) healing for Mike

Pray for secondary infections.

Pray for all illnesses. People pass in this hospital every day. Let it always make us respect life and it's fragility

Quotes for today:

"The way I see it- if you want the rainbow you must put up with the rain."

"Don't wait until you reach your goal to be proud of yourself. Be proud of every step you take."

"It's always the small pieces that make the big picture."

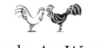

Steady As We Go.

"Life's battles don't always go to the stronger or faster man. But sooner or later, the man who wins is the man who thinks he can."

As always:

Beat the bumps

Let go and let God.

If you ain't cheatin, you ain't tryin.

steady as we go

Love Sarah

Scripture:

Isaiah 41:13, For I am the Lord your God, who takes hold of your right hand and says to you, do not fear; I will help you.

Reflection:

Sometimes the most courageous thing that we can do, is to stop trying to do it all on our own. It is hard to release a loved one to God, but it is the best thing that we can do. We do not have the power to heal, but God does and there is so much wisdom in letting go and letting God. No, only can He fix the broken things in our lives, but He wants to. He just wants you to ask and believe. Believe with a mustard seed of faith. Pray and give it to your father in heaven and it will be done.

Author Sarah VanNetten

THE LESSONS OF PAIN

Day 56/ June 2ⁿᵈ

Every day spent in the ICU is a day that I see Mike getting stronger. I can see his personality coming through, his memory is spot on. He knows what is happening, he wants to get better. He wants to be stronger. I love watching him learn to communicate with all his people... his arm motions, his animation, his smiles, and fist pumps. Today he asked me why he can't talk... Caught me off guard. I'm sure he has been told, but I told him he has a trach in his throat, (which he knows) but with the air being blown in and the air needed to speak, it is just a whisper right now... Don't worry Mikey, it will come back to you. Hoping they can downsize his trach and he can have a speaking valve attached. He does get frustrated, but he is getting better at it and realized we won't stop till we get what he wants to say. For all that Mike has had thrown at him, some of which he has no idea, he just keeps making these steps toward his goal. Has this been easy for anyone... not! Why do bad things happen to the best of people? Why does pain exist in our world? Pain, it gets our attention, it helps us to focus on what really matters in life. What is important, (I know this to be true). Pain helps to develop character. My good friend Ann sends me a devotion every morning so for this next statement I can take no credit, but it needs to be said, so think about it. Pain gives us two choices, the first is to be bitter and angry and to let it eat you. The second is to learn from it. Almost everything that enhances and enlightens your conscience comes through affliction. Suffering helps you to be more gracious, understanding, humble. You are more vulnerable to others and their feelings (true)! This event has transformed and

Steady As We Go.

changed Mike, me, our family, and I dare say some of you...we can't help but be and live and feel differently. Pain increases our ability to help others., put ourselves in their shoes. If we don't look for the good, the bad is all-consuming and both the pain and Satan wins. I think this makes sense (thanks Ann). "If suffering can be used for the greater good, if it's a means to develop character, then it is plausible that a loving God would allow pain. Pain and a loving God can co-exist." Mini sermon for tonight, but pain exists in this world... use it to our benefit and good.

So here is what I learned about my Mikey, your Mike, your Chicken today. Mike had a good night's sleep. He is now sitting in his chair for an hour a morning. He talks every day about how damn good that popsicle was, but he was not quite ready... not yet Mike, have your thickened apple juice for now... soon! Ally is Mike's nurse today. We had her in the early days, Mike does not remember, but she is thrilled to have him over here. She has a lot of energy, and she is excited that Mike is going outside again today. These people always ask me what it is like outside? They don't get out in a workday, so she is almost as excited as Mike to sit outside for a while. First physio with Michelle today. Stronger everyday. Whereas we used to need a nurse, 2 physio and a respiratory therapist to do a walk, we are down to a nurse and a physio. Today Mike again walked farther, he keeps beating himself. He is amazing! Then outside. Another beautiful day and he got to visit with his dad, his brother and Cindy. He was so happy to see them. It's tough, the goodbye is tough, but it's not goodbye, never say that word, it is seeing you soon. Mike is caught up on crops and farm and friends and then it's time to go in... His dad says, so soon?... Yep, oxygen tank is almost empty, our time is up! Fair enough. Love to everyone, strength until our next visit. Mike went back up for more chair time, another 40 min. We did a Facetime with our new Ireland Road farmer, Farmer Walker and saw his local operation. Mike smiled the whole time. When we were wrapping up, they were taking their son Mikey for his vaccine... they said he was nervous... Mike mouthed, and it was clear to see, 'Get it, you don't want to be me'... damn you don't. Mike is a lucky one, luck isn't even a word. What he is, is a miracle brought through by prayer, the knowledge and gift God gave to these people, and Mike's sheer determination... so no you don't ever want to be here... eating from a tube in your nose to your stomach and breathing from a trach in your neck and being denied a simple pleasure of a popsicle for the fear that it may go into your lungs. It was great to talk to the Walkers. Adam assured Mike that this chicken farming after helping Ryan for a day isn't nearly as hard as Mike has made it out to be... when he gets home, Adam will treat Mike to a day of banking to see how real people work.

When I left Mike was resting in bed. Nurse Ally was just coming back from coffee. He was going to watch the Jays tonight. Tomorrow is a new day, full of new possibilities, new goals, new steps to home. When I got home from the hospital the most beautiful bouquet of flowers was waiting at home... from Mike... he asked his dad to get it for me "Thanks for all you have done."

.. It was for us and our family Mike, there is too much left to do. See you tomorrow!

Individual prayer requests

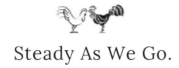

Steady As We Go.

For complete restoration of Mike's health

Secondary infections be kept far away

For doctors and nurses' knowledge… they are truly learning every day… there is limited research… Mike is their research

For all patients suffering and recovering

Quotes for today:

"A bird sitting on a tree is never afraid of the branch breaking because its trust is not in the branch, but in its own wings. Always believe in yourself."

"The best feeling in the world is finally knowing you took a step in the right direction. A step towards the future where everything that you never thought was possible is possible."

"Everything is coming together. Stay positive, patient, and trust the timing of your life."

As always:

beat the bumps,

Let go and let God.

If you ain't cheatin, you ain't tryin

Steady as we go

Love Sarah

Scripture:

Psalm 46:10, Cease striving and know that I am God; I will be exalted among the nations, I will be exalted in the earth.

Reflection:

Relax in my healing, holy presence. Let go of your cares and your worries, was my devotion for day 56. Do not get so wrapped up in yourself and what is happening to you that you lose sight of Me! Good advice. … this is another reason that I am a believer because right when I needed to hear something, I heard it. I don't believe it was a coincidence or an aligning of the stars but that I was sent what I needed to get through the day. Relax … become less tense and anxious. Relax… become less tense in my anxiety, don't be anxious. Such tall words for mine or what situation you may be facing. But what control did I have, do any of us have over our situations. There are days and weeks I could have buried myself in fear and anxiety, many face the same turmoil in their lives for different reasons. So, I suppose my lesson today is to relax… breathe… find a faith, an anchor, a way to get through what demon you face. You will never accomplish anything on your own.

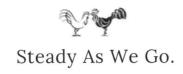

Steady As We Go.

PATIENCE FOR PATIENTS

Day 57/ June 3rd

New life, new norm. It's amazing how quickly you adapt to a new routine, whether you like it or not. School still will remain online, (honestly happy cause no lunches). My oldest Zack works at Canadian Tire and starts at 5:30am ... he does enjoy a long shower so 4:30 is the wake-up time, ... I got up with Mike when he was working and left the house at 5 am. I put his lunch in his pail and then into his hand to get him out the door. I am not going to not do it for the son that is so clearly yours! Anyway, off Zack goes and I get about my day. You would think you would get a lot done at that time in the morning, but less than one would think.

If I have learned anything during this time it is the art of patience. God bless patience...Patience is not my forte. Think about it... patience does not come naturally, often we are too impatient to develop it. The control is taken out of our hands, and I LOVE CONTROL. I love having control and I love having patience if it gets me what I want... then I can be patient. I love organizing, I hate surprises, I like to have fun, but on my terms and in my ways, then I am super fun. I was the queen of university fun. I loved to go out, but on my control and to the level of my patience, I hated waiting... Many is the night waiting to go out for the night, and everyone would be having a drink and a good time, I would think it was time to go... they would say no Sarah, we have lots of time... 5 minutes later, I would announce, "Cab is here friends! Time to go!!" Eye roll from everyone, but off we would go... and most times to avoid the bar line up I might add. I love control, and if you have control, you at some point have patience, because things go your way.

Here, not so much. I have no control, so I must have the patience. I have learned, patience, in situations, leads to trusting God, giving him control... who else can I turn to? I can honestly say, I had faith before, but my faith has grown each day. It is stronger. Think about it... patients, and patience are homophones, but I can't help but think how patients may, possess the patience to get them through.

This is what I learned today about my Mikey, your Mike, your Chicken today. This day makes me smile. Mike is amazing... he truly is. He had a decent sleep last night. Thank you. I am so thankful to be spending more time with Mike. My kids are good at home, their housekeeping skills are to be desired but...

When I arrived, Mike is lying in bed, gown up to go in, so happy to see him, he is trying to tell me something, so animated with his hands, wiping his forehead, pointing under the bed, I look under the bed, there is a stool. I get it, he is tired, physio Michelle was in this morning, she had him doing the step stool with his walker, up and down, he is wiped-out but damn... so good. Speech therapist Alannah comes in to talk and she is happy. We all realize the popsicle was a disaster, but Mike would do it over and over to feel that beautiful feel. The other good news is that respiratory therapist, Jennifer downsized his trach, so if that goes well over the weekend, Mike will have a new X-ray to see how his swallow goes. Thumbs up. Jennifer comes back in and says ok Mike... next trick, smaller trach... puts on the speaking valve...Mike has a strong whisper. I am so proud, I am so

Steady As We Go.

happy, eye leak, eye leak. My gosh, I just don't have words. No time though, get your workout socks on ... time to go. Michelle walks in... Mike... 'Hi Michelle." Double take... MIKE! It's a whisper, but it is amazing. Ally is his nurse again today, he really likes her, as do I. It is Ally and Alyson double-teaming in the room today, couldn't be happier. Michelle comes back in the room for afternoon workout. Mike gets up better on his own, he is stronger. He goes farther. Mike has a halfway rest in his chair to recover. Some nurses he has had pass by and Mike whispers... " I am on my way out! ".. they are so sure he is soon. He is loved up here. He walks back to the room and passes a cleaning lady who has pulled to the side to let Mike pass, he looks at her and smiles and says, "Beat you." Oh, my Mikey. Back to chair time. He is so tired but so proud. So am I. He is too tired to Face Time. Just get through the chair time which he does, then back to bed. We talked a bit. His whisper will get stronger, every day. For now know, Mike remembers going to Norfolk General back on April 8th. He knows (it's important to him) that Angie Miller gave him ginger ale... something special Angie. He knows that once he had an X-ray their concern was great. More will come, but he is grateful, he knows where he was, and he remembers the love taps... don't ever think that people in a coma state cannot hear you... do not ever give up. Where there is life there is hope. Never doubt. Never lose faith or hope. Believe, trust God, pray.

    I leave you with this...as Mike is lying back in bed we are whispering, and I can hear Colton's dad playing music, I recognize some songs, a Travis Tritt, another one, and then I hear The Gambler... suddenly Mike's eyes look at me and he is pointing at the curtain, his eyes are going wide, and I am ... yes... The Gambler. Mike. Then, and I will see this forever in my head, starts moving his feet and his hand is hitting the mattress and he in his most powerful whisper sings the words. My gosh. my thoughts, I did not ruin this song for him by singing it to him all the time... I look at him, there is joy in his face, he looks like Mike singing his song and I quietly chime in on the chorus.

Love you Mike, I will see you tomorrow. As I leave, I tell Colton's dad how much we loved his music and especially The Gambler... The 2 of us have shed many tears between our curtains. After hearing of Mike's love of The Gambler, Colton's dad tells me he will play it louder next time! Prayers for Mike, for Colton and for Kansas City Brad tonight... and prayers for anyone who needs them. Storm heaven for everyone!!

Individual prayer requests:

Complete healing for Mike and other Covid patients.

For secondary infections to be far away

For these amazing health care workers. Health care includes the people who disinfect or ensure garbage is changed so no infection can travel

Pray for our world

Quotes for tonight:

"Patience with others is love."

"Patience with self is hope."

"Patience with God is faith."

Steady As We Go.

happy, eye leak, eye leak. My gosh, I just don't have words. No time though, get your workout socks on … time to go. Michelle walks in… Mike… 'Hi Michelle." Double take… MIKE! It's a whisper, but it is amazing. Ally is his nurse again today, he really likes her, as do I. It is Ally and Alyson double-teaming in the room today, couldn't be happier. Michelle comes back in the room for afternoon workout. Mike gets up better on his own, he is stronger. He goes farther. Mike has a halfway rest in his chair to recover. Some nurses he has had pass by and Mike whispers… " I am on my way out! ".. they are so sure he is soon. He is loved up here. He walks back to the room and passes a cleaning lady who has pulled to the side to let Mike pass, he looks at her and smiles and says, "Beat you." Oh, my Mikey. Back to chair time. He is so tired but so proud. So am I. He is too tired to Face Time. Just get through the chair time which he does, then back to bed. We talked a bit. His whisper will get stronger, every day. For now know, Mike remembers going to Norfolk General back on April 8th. He knows (it's important to him) that Angie Miller gave him ginger ale… something special Angie. He knows that once he had an X-ray their concern was great. More will come, but he is grateful, he knows where he was, and he remembers the love taps… don't ever think that people in a coma state cannot hear you… do not ever give up. Where there is life there is hope. Never doubt. Never lose faith or hope. Believe, trust God, pray.

    I leave you with this…as Mike is lying back in bed we are whispering, and I can hear Colton's dad playing music, I recognize some songs, a Travis Tritt, another one, and then I hear The Gambler… suddenly Mike's eyes look at me and he is pointing at the curtain, his eyes are going wide, and I am ... yes... The Gambler. Mike. Then, and I will see this forever in my head, starts moving his feet and his hand is hitting the mattress and he in his most powerful whisper sings the words. My gosh. my thoughts, I did not ruin this song for him by singing it to him all the time... I look at him, there is joy in his face, he looks like Mike singing his song and I quietly chime in on the chorus.

Love you Mike, I will see you tomorrow. As I leave, I tell Colton's dad how much we loved his music and especially The Gambler... The 2 of us have shed many tears between our curtains. After hearing of Mike's love of The Gambler, Colton's dad tells me he will play it louder next time! Prayers for Mike, for Colton and for Kansas City Brad tonight... and prayers for anyone who needs them. Storm heaven for everyone!!

Individual prayer requests:

Complete healing for Mike and other Covid patients.

For secondary infections to be far away

For these amazing health care workers. Health care includes the people who disinfect or ensure garbage is changed so no infection can travel

Pray for our world

Quotes for tonight:

"Patience with others is love."

"Patience with self is hope."

"Patience with God is faith."

Steady As We Go.

"It always rains the hardest on the people that deserve the sun."

"Never give up on something that you-can't go a day without thinking about."

"No matter how you feel: get up, dress up, show up and never give up."

As always:

Beat the bumps Mikey

let go and let God.

if you ain't cheatin you ain't tryin

Steady as we go.

Love, Sarah

Scripture:

Jeremiah 31:25, I will refresh the weary and satisfy the faint

Reflections:

      My heart hurts for those who are still suffering this virus. My heart still hurts for the messages I receive daily from those who's loved one has just been ventilated or whose situation has worsened. My heart aches for the length of recovery, the unknown still ahead. My eyes tear for those of whom I now consider friends who go another day to the hospital to encourage or sit with their loved one. I feel lucky... but some days still so sad. I want everyone to beat this. I want everyone to BELIEVE this. It angers me those who speak so casually about it, or God forbid it is something made up. How can you argue with science??

I am so happy to see people on the beach, planning a next year, trying to resume a normal life. The whole reason I have a story to tell... one I never wanted to. I will never forget because of Covid. It still exists. Please be diligent, please don't think it couldn't be you. Give health care the respect they deserve. Please be vaccinated.

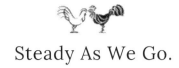

Steady As We Go.

MOVING ON UP

Day 58/ June 4th

Fifty-eight days of being in hospital... a quick and vital diagnosis from our Norfolk General Hospital here in Simcoe was critical for Mike. Thank heavens for their realization of his situation and for a speedy move to Burlington. A few days in Burlington, Mike was ventilated and then again, a realization that more was needed, a chance to go on ECMO at The Hamilton General... and that is where we have been since. For now... this is home. The 3rd floor ICU has been our home for 54 days. They have seen Mike from one end of the hallway, through 4 room changes... which brought him to the other end of the hallway. This is where Mike went from having his back against the wall. a few times, to the day he NEEDED to start making baby steps and he did! To the progression of getting off ECMO, dialysis, to removing a breathing tube and replacing it with a trach. From going from ventilated oxygen to hi flow. From having his physio girls in the early days just simply moving limbs quietly, to this morning, Yvonne, Yvonne, taking Mike downstairs to a stairwell and doing 2 steps up, 2 steps down, 2 steps up, 2 steps down. This is the home that has cheered him on, celebrated him, has come to look at him and say to him. "I had you in the early days when you were very ill... you won't remember me, but I just wanted to come and see you and to say how proud and happy we are." Today there was a transport into the adjoining room, and I recognize nurse

Andre wheeling the patient in. I say to Mike's nurse today Allana ... that is Andre, isn't it? She said "Yes that is him, he is so funny". I agree with her 100 percent. Mike looks at us and asks, "Who is Andre?" Mike is only getting to know these amazing people now. I tell him Andre was your nurse a couple times in the early days, and he would spend his time charting inside your room so he could talk sports to you. I loved him. I am not normally a names person... they exit my mind as quickly as they enter, but I have tried during these days especially hard to remember names, to be able to call by name whenever I can. As Mike says he doesn't remember many of these people, I do... I know what they did. They have a name and deserve recognition.

So here is what I learned today about my Mikey, your Mike, your Chicken. Today is another great day. Real steps in the morning. Confidence in doing them. When I arrived shortly afternoon. Mike's voice is so much louder! An adjustment to the voice attachment and it's like wow!! Way beyond a whisper. He says don't get comfortable; we are moving. Leaving ICU, headed to '8th-floor medicine.' Non surgery floor. So wonderful! Amazing news! The move is in the works, but physio will not be dismissed so here comes Yvonne, Yvonne. Time to walk, she is just amazing, they all are, but she has this fire of energy, with the best accent. She tells Mike she will be checking in on him on 8 and that she is sending up the hardest program... wouldn't expect less. After Mike's walk with Yvonne, we went outside with nurse Allana. The double W's were visitors, Walker and Woody and it was great. Mike's voice is stronger. I love watching him with his friends. They are all in agreement that it is lucky he was 'robust' to start with and he had 45 pounds to lose... he would have faded away to nothing.... eye roll eye, roll by me. Oxygen tank almost out, see you soon, can't wait to be home.

Steady As We Go.

Back inside and loading to go... Mike does not have a lot of possessions here, he has pictures and toiletries, but he has some equipment to come along. Ok, how do I sum this up... leaving this floor, this 'home' was emotional, this was our family, our people away from our people at home. This was our comfort zone, our safe. This was the place "where everybody knows your name"...

Cousin Chris Misner is working today and in the room, as we prepare to leave, what can I say, how can I thank you for being Mike's biggest advocate, for being there for me, I can't ... and I know you want nothing but what you have done for us, it can never be put into words... and between you and your red headed friend, and ECMO man and everyone else you call your work family. I thank you from the depths of my soul. You all wear your scrubs and walk those halls as angels. eye leak, hug, eternal thanks.

New home, for now, is the 8th floor. I have talked a lot for tonight. Mike is on 8 now. He will remain where he is for a few days to monitor him then will receive a new room on this floor until he can go to rehab... but I don't feel that is far off. I really don't. This floor is unfamiliar, but Mike makes friends everywhere... and I tell you this. ...As Mike's nurse Allana from 3 was passing the binder off to his new nurse on 8, I heard their conversation and it was, new nurse said, I started my research on who the new patient is, and it is the hospital famous guy... not only in this hospital, but Ontario famous guy. Alanna replied, yes this is him. I stayed longer to be sure he was ok... and as he is talking to his nurse and doctor they say, what a story you have had, his response is yes, and I am starting to write my last few pages so let's keep going.

I can't even think of how to end this tonight other than believe in yourself and maybe have a little faith in what you think you can't do, because I am pretty sure we are all capable of a little bit more. Pain is temporary… It gets you to where you want to be.

Individual prayer requests:

Pray for a settlement for Mike onto floor 8. For his calm and assurance.

Pray for a new swallow test on Monday or Tuesday and that the feeding tube can be removed… the man needs a popsicle and some chicken nuggets and fries

I can tell you I receive so many sad stories about others suffering, and I ask you to pray for all those struggling, mentally, physically, emotionally… God is capable of all.

Pray for doctors and nurses on all floors

Quotes for Tonight:

"Beautiful pictures are developed from negatives in a dark room… so if you see darkness in your life, be reassured that a beautiful picture is being prepared."

"Keep going because you didn't come this far to only come this far."

"Give yourself some credit for the days you made it when you thought you couldn't."

"Start by doing what is necessary, then do what's possible: and suddenly you are doing the impossible."

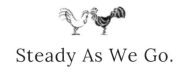

Steady As We Go.

As always:

Beat the bumps Mikey

let go and let God

If you ain't cheatin you ain't tryin

Steady as we go

Love Sarah

Scripture:

1 Chronicles 16:11, Look to the Lord and his strength; seek his face always.

Reflection:

One day the mountain that is in front of you will be so far behind you, it will barely be visible in the distance. But the person you became learning to get over it? That will stay with you forever- AND THAT, is the point of the **mountain!**

LAZY SATURDAY

Day 59 /June 5th

First full day up here on 8th floor medicine. A basically whole new world. 2 nurses for 4 patients. I can't wait to meet these people on 8th. These next couple of days are about monitoring. Kinda unexciting, but necessary. His night nurse was excellent and said that he settled in just fine. The day nurse is Rachelle… there is another, but Rachelle is his main. Mike finally has a call button. The nurses sit in a window facing his bed. Two roommates across from him. He has a locker to put his toiletries in. To be honest. I really have no new update today… it is the weekend; physio doesn't happen up here as it does in ICU… Mike moved from his bed to his chair several times. He has excellent nurses and excellent doctors up here. He had a doctor from the RACE team (I hope I got the right initials) come and check on him from ICU. There is a constant writing in that binder that is Mike. But until Monday… we are kinda in a stagnation… a waiting period. He has not needed neck suction, nor has he suctioned his own mouth. Today was uneventful, I am bored on a Saturday afternoon, nothing to do day. (You know what, after the last 58 days, not so bad). I don't want Mike to have a rest day… but I get how it is important to move him to the next step.

So here is what I learned today about my Mikey your Mike your Chicken. We all know Chicken is a fighter. This is not the floor where people are turning cartwheels and sitting around the table eating dinners. We are still in life-threatening injuries. These are sad cases. So as much as we have moved forward, it is crazy/sad to see. So, this is what I

Steady As We Go.

want to say. Mike is so grateful for his life. He gets that every step is a step closer to home. There is work ahead, he just wants to get at it. Sadness sucks. It sucks when anyone experiences it, so it is sad to come to a room where 2 more people are experiencing sadness.

Mike amazes me with his attitude, his determination... well he amazes me every day, he will succeed in his goal. Cousin Chris came up on break. As weird as it is, Mike misses them, and they miss him... she says you can't count the people that have stopped by to see him, and "He is on to the 8th". I hope Colton joins us soon! Mike misses him too.

Something to think about how our lives can change in an instant, leaving us or those we love in circumstances that feel impossible to bear. Tomorrow cannot be taken for granted, 5 minutes from now cannot be taken for granted. But when we are willing to share all God has given us, in my opinion, my feelings, my trust, my hope in his healing... while we wait on him, we can hold onto his love. Without that, I am not sure what I would have done. I know that Mike would not be where he is without the love of God and prayers that were fervent and constant.

Mike is looking forward to next week... anxiously awaiting. We know he has a swallowing test early in the week... he wants to pass. This is the next step. He is not hungry but craving a taste... guess what... McDonald's chicken nuggets and fries (supporting the industry). Slow patient steps, adapting to a new environment, temporary stop, bring on rehab. Patience, patience, patience.

Mike, I know, "You had this the whole time."

Individual prayer requests,

Pray for complete healing for Mike.

I pray for a speedy move through floor 8

I pray for all those on this floor, there are so many different things they are addressing, and it is not happiness always

Quotes for today,

"Success comes when you simply refuse to give up- with goals so strong that obstacles only act as motivation."

"Instead of waiting for the storm to pass, dance your way through it."

"Every beautiful thing in the world is rooted in some sort of pain."

As always,

beat the bumps Mikey

Let go and let God.

If you ain't cheatin, you ain't tryin

Steady as we go

Love Sarah

Scripture: Romans 12:12, Be joyful in hope, patient in affliction, faithful in prayer.

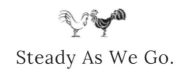

Steady As We Go.

Reflection:

Steady as we go. From early on this has become our go-to saying. It was and is so perfect. My cousin Chris used it when she was always talking to me on the phone. She would say it several times in all the conversations. The day I called to tell her Mike was coming to the General to be put on ECMO she said to me, "Now you are entering my world." She knew what that world was all about and yes, be steady as we go through it. Stay as calm as you can, you will get through it.

Applies still to life. It is so easy to get worked up about things and anxious, worry can take over and worry usually leads to fear. Deep breath and remember … steady as we go!

Author Sarah VanNetten

STEADY SUNDAY

Day 60/ June 6th

Here we are back to another Sunday... God's extra day of work on Mike's behalf. Mike's bad days have fallen on Sundays more times than I care to remember. Last night when I left the hospital Mike and I talked about Sundays and he said, I am done with bad days... tomorrow will be a good Sunday. He has held his promise. This has been a beautiful Sunday!

This morning we welcomed a new calf to the farm who was born sometime in the night. Moodonna did the job all on her own and gave birth to a beautiful girl cow (I am sure a girl cow has another name, but I have only been a calf owner for 12 hours now). This is really another miracle. A year and a half ago we got 2 young cows to grow for beef, a male and female. The male we used for what we intended. The female we waited on as we didn't have the cooler room at the time... then Mike got sick and Moodonna was the luckiest cow in the world to just keep grazing... luckily because until recently we didn't know she was pregnant. If Mike had not gotten sick, she and her young one's fate would have been much different. Taku (bull) managed to get his work done and today Moodonna became a mom to Steady Sunday. We all know where the name, Steady came from... and Sunday is just perfect (Thank you, Jen). Sunday because Mike will have a good one. Today is also a special day for us as it would have been Mike's mom, Tina's 69th birthday. A special gift from heaven above today. Not only did she push Mike back to us, but she sent a calf to say that she loves us and here is something happy to have on my first birthday without me. Tina always loved her birthday, so this is truly an amazing

Steady As We Go.

gift. I know how much we are all missing her today, always just a thought away. Welcome Steady Sunday to the farm.

I will admit, I can now add to the resume, with Ryan's help, putting a calf up to her mom to drink for the first time, and I now know how to start milk flow on a cow... Steady Sunday became busy drinking! I also can admit that calf raising, for the time being, is over my head- so with a check-up this morning from our good friend Blake Pow, we all have agreed that Moodonna and Steady Sunday will go live with another cow friend, Andrew Phibbs for the first month to ensure all goes well. These cows are part of this story. I want the best for them!

Here is what I learned about my Mikey, your Mike, and your Chicken today. Mike once again had a good night. They were able to move him to the minimal settings on his oxygen. There were several Face Times from the barn this morning so he could see the happenings. Mike is a huge animal lover, so he is so excited. I wish he could have been here... but soon enough. For now, all is under control. When I arrive, Mike is laying in bed talking on the phone... all this work is sure to improve his swallow skills as well. He also got physio this morning... (thank you Yvonne, Yvonne) for your persistence... you speak, and people listen. Mike walked with one of his new physio men and his walker all around the block of his ward. He was so happy he did it well! Even Mike was worried about a day of rest (this must be a new Mike... so focused on his exercise!) The staff up here is amazing too. Doctor Brittany is part of the team, and she is so pleased. Mike jokes with them, they laugh, he says enjoy me now because I am out of here! They have a hope to cork his trach today, she says... she will write up the order and a respiratory therapist will be in to do it. So, at 2:30 Mike had his trach corked and he is now breathing completely his own. 100% his own air. There is nose oxygen available at any time if his oxygen goes down, or simply uncork and put back on hi-flow. It is not unusual to use oxygen during the nights, but so far so good. We will see how this trial goes. Might I just say again... he makes me so proud. I know this is hard work. Learning to breath again. Being confident when you are there by yourself, knowing that not a real life, but life is happening outside these windows, and you are inside... the reason you are doing the work is to get to this outside world. To see the life that exists outside these walls however feeble it may be right now. My devotion today was this... my world is full of beautiful things, they are meant to be pointers to me, reminders of God's abiding presence. I don't need to look very far... only to see that my calf was born on a Sunday, which was also Tina's birthday. I saw it in the sunset last night on my drive home, I see it in Mike's smile and his determination. I see it in the people who he talks with or Face Times with who say to me, he hasn't missed a beat, he is Mike, he is funny, he asks about you... he may be 50 pounds lighter, but he is Mike... Yes, he is.

So, to wrap up, we hope this week Mike gets to a wardroom and very soon, a rehab facility. We hope that this trach can be removed as soon as possible, and we hope that Mike passes with flying colors his swallow test. I believe that all these are done deals... but I also know that I am not in control, but God is. So, I hope for these, and I put it in God's hands. When I last talked to Mike on the phone basically to discuss our new cow operation, Mike was in great spirits. He had spoken to a few people on the phone, he was going to

Steady As We Go.

watch some iPad and get ready for sleep. At first, I know I was the one that spoke on his behalf... I was the encourager for Mike... but I truly feel he is encouraging me now. I am so proud of him and his work, his desire. We will be normal again sometime soon... our whole world will be... in the meantime, do your part... wear the mask, get your vaccination, book your second if you can. Thank an angel in scrubs and let's please get ready to have some fun again... together, all vaccinated and safe to live what life truly does have to offer us. It's within our reach.

Individual prayer requests:

Pray for the corking of Mike's trach and for his swallow test.

Pray for continued strength as he learns to breathe again

Pray for all those suffering whatever unknown illness that may be

Pray for these health care workers... they are brilliant

Quotes for tonight:

"We are to savour God and his great deeds in the little moments of our everyday."

"Let your strongest muscle be your will."

"The struggle is real, but so are the blessings."

"Wake up."

"Be kind."

"Kick ass."

"Repeat!"

As always:

beat the bumps Mikey

Let go and let God

If you ain't cheatin you ain't tryin

Steady as we go.

Love Sarah

Scripture:

Psalm 19: 1-2, The heavens declare the glory of God; the skies proclaim the work of his hands. Day after day they pour forth speech, night after night they display knowledge.

Reflection:

The world is full of beautiful things that are meant to be pointers to God and reminders of his presence. The skies proclaim the works of his hands. It is natural to become frustrated and it is a real world where doubt creeps in. That is where this verse speaks to me and is so reassuring. The skies sing of God. The stars in the night sky when you look up, how can you not see God's hand in that sky. A sunset with so many brilliant colours that looks like it was painted... I see that and I see a reminder that God is with us always. Beautiful things that point us towards God, ask us to pause for a moment and remember his greatness. In a world where it sometimes seems it can be out of control; God puts these reminders in our path ... for these I am so grateful.

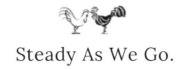
Steady As We Go.

GIVE IT TO GOD

Day 61/ June 7th

    If there is one thing, I think I have always struggled with in life, it is worry. Although I feel I handle it much better, I have always thought of myself as a worry wart. I have always worried about having the friends I wanted, I worried about what they would think of me. I always worried about my grades and studying and how I was going to do in tests. I worried as I said the other day about such silly things as whether we would have to wait in lineups to get into pubs. I remember always calling my dad after driving me back to school to be sure he arrived home safe. I think I LOVED worrying… This is the best thing, I met and married the most laid back, happy, pleasing person you have ever met. Mike does not worry about who likes him, what he wears, (who doesn't love his multi purpose everyday go anywhere shoes). He doesn't worry about what you think of him, or money, or what is for supper. He just takes life as it is. Maybe that is due to circumstances he has come across in life and has come out on the better side and as a stronger person. Maybe it is because he sees life for the gift it is. Maybe it is that in his heart of hearts he knows that people admire all these qualities in him and are drawn to him. They want just a bit of his sparkle.

    This is a big couple days for Mike, with his swallow test tomorrow, (I only share this because we welcome prayers for it). It is kinda like your driving test when you are 16, you don't want to tell anyone you went until you went there and passed. He has also had his trach corked for over 24 beautiful hours as well, he is mostly breathing room oxygen.

Today Mike is worried about tomorrow, so I told him this. My most favorite bible verse is Matthew 6:27, Who by worrying can add a single hour to his life. Matthew 6:35, Therefore do not worry about tomorrow for tomorrow will worry about itself, each day has enough trouble of its own. My devotion this morning was entitled 'worry'. It said the following. Who oversees your life? If it, is you (yourself), then you have good reason to worry? But since it is I AM (God), in charge, worry is both unnecessary and counterproductive. God will take care of the problem or show you how to handle it period. Or maybe a bit of both. I read this to Mike today and said, every time tonight you get a bit worried, push it aside and say a prayer instead.

So here is what I learned about my Mikey, your Mike, your Chicken today. Mike is making strides. He wants home in the worst way but knows it isn't time. Today our hay was baled by friends. Our cows were picked up by friends... Mike is so grateful to friends... if someone else were in this room, he would be the first out there to help, but now to accept... thank you. The bailers were more than happy. Mike we are drinking your beer!

Mike is gaining strength every day. Sitting in the chair a bit more often. He can walk a short distance without any support at all besides a nurse walking beside him in case. He had physio today, and some more bed exercises to focus on his breathing inhale in, breath in the coffee, exhale out, blow out the candles. Mix your exercises with working your lungs. Deep breaths. Mike is practicing. Almost done... Rachel, was a wonderful nurse today. They are getting the chance to see

Steady As We Go.

Mike's personality and although there are some sad moments, on both our sides… there is no where else I want to be these days. Steady as we go. So much ahead of us. Every time Mike talks to anyone, his last sentence is, we are going to have one party when I am home and allowed… not right away, but eventually. I just can't wait. Also, Chris Misner and Bob Mehlenbacher, the Whisley club will be ringing the bell.

Individual Prayer requests:

Complete restoration of health to Mike …body, soul, mind.

Peace of mind for the cork of the trach and his swallow test.

I pray for this floor, so many different cases, from seizures, to palliative to addictions… so many needs for prayer and healing.

As always for all the people working in this amazing building.

Quotes for today:

"Be like the ocean. Breathtaking to look at, strong enough not to be destroyed and gentle enough so others find comfort in your presence."

"Whenever you find yourself doubting how far you can go just remember how far you have come. Remember everything you have faced, all the battles you have won, and all the fears you have overcome."

"A little more persistence, a little more effort, and what seemed hopeless failure may turn to glorious success."

As always:

Beat the bumps the Mikey

Let go and let God.

If you ain't cheatin you ain't tryin

Steady as we go

Love Sarah

Scripture:

Matthew 6:27, Who of you by worrying can add a single hour to his life?

Reflection:

I love what I said …. every time tonight you get a little bit worried, push it aside and say a prayer instead. Sometimes I really need to take my own advice. I still worry. I find it hard not to. It's not home and life is normal. … life is good but it's a different normal and I worry about Mike. I worry about his strength, I worry about his meds, I worry about the humid air and his lungs, I worry what his long-term effects of Covid will be … and the list goes on. Why though? Worry is natural but it leads to nothing good, and it clearly says it can add no hours to your life. If anything worry shortens our lives. It's also true if God cares so much for the birds of the air, how much more love he has for us… so what is the point in the worry. So, friends who have lately witnessed my worry, I am going to try harder. When the worries come, I'm going to pause and say a prayer. It works. I have felt God take my worry and give me peace instead. To worry over things, you aren't even sure will happen is a waste of this beautiful life we have been gifted. See the blessings, let God do the worrying.

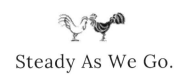
Steady As We Go.

Author Sarah VanNetten

THE GOUT

Day 62/ June 8th

April 8, 2021... the day I dropped Mike to NGH scared, but confident that I had not misdiagnosed his man cold (I only say this as I will never ever use that phrase again, I will never deny a gut feeling that I know that I ignored... because I thought that he would be better tomorrow). I am eternally grateful that Mike asked to go to the hospital that day as I am pretty sure we would not be sitting where we are if I had waited even hours more. So, this is where we stand two months later. Two months of some rock bottom downs and some most amazing ups. From listening to our doctors and remembering to never get too excited in either step forward or backward steps... steady as we go. Now here we are, and I am just so happy to be able to tell you of Mike's progress that he has made on his two-month anniversary of being a patient of our amazing medical system.

So here is what I learned today about my Mikey, your Mike, and your Chicken. For all those who know Mike, they know in the past he has suffered from 'the gout'. The gout according to Mike has always been caused by the asparagus I forced on his plate... nothing to do with the beverages that accompanied the one sprig... but it was the sprig. Apparently and according to Mike, possibly the worst thing a person could ever suffer from.... forget about childbirth, have you ever had a sheet touch your toe while having the gout? No??? Then you have no idea the pain I am experiencing. Be happy you birthed children without pain meds, this is brutal. Well last night the gout struck Mike... and I did not feed him

Steady As We Go.

asparagus, and they put none in his feed tube... just sayin. Anyway, we know Mike has been through unbelievable pain these past days, but he said last night he was in tears with the pain. The team finally diagnosed him with gout and hopefully have him on the proper meds. I will add this in... as I know Mike is reading...when my cousin Chris popped in, without Mike saying, she said, yes Greg (her husband) has gotten gout too and he gets it from asparagus. Mike looked at her and shed a tear... did you hear that, Sarah! someone who believes me. Asparagus causes gout! Eye roll eye roll by me... Yes, Mike you never have to eat asparagus again. Ok gout was the bad part of Mike's Day. Swallow test at 9 this morning. Mike passed. He passed everything except he is not allowed straws. We can live with that. I wanted to head down right away so I left home at 10 to see Mike.

When I arrive, his respiratory therapist is in the room with him, they wanted it to be a surprise, but we are taking Mike's trach out! This is amazing news!! Oh my, so then and there they take out his trach, and cover it with a band-aid and it should close within 48 hours. To watch him sit and touch that band-aid after and to not quite believe it... and to see if his voice still worked and to check if he could still breathe without it. My gosh this is amazing. He is beyond grateful. I am beyond grateful. He will receive lunch today! That kinda got mixed up and lunch didn't arrive. We know he can eat anything except carrots and celery. perfect I hate them anyways. So, I went to the cafe and looked around and got Mike a little bistro pizza and a butter tart. That was his first food, a slice of pizza and a butter tart, his most favourite treat. After his lunch physio, Debbie came in. Unfortunately, the gout has bound him to the bed for the day, but no worries, she did fantastic bed exercises and she brought bands and she worked on his breathing with room air. His yoga breathing is coming along. Debbie is a fellow Dutch girl as well and she is lovely.

More great news... Mike has been in medicine step down... he is moving to a wardroom and for now it will be a single room. It is amazing. Mike says goodbye to Joe, who is Kim's husband who lays in the bed across from Mike. They have become chummy these past couple days and each night joe goes home and has a beer for Mike, and everyone else who can't. Kim is not well so she as well needs prayers. So many are up here. His old nurse Liz passes him off to his new nurse Vanessa and Vanessa is mentoring Victoria who has just finished school and his starting her orientation. She is young and enthusiastic and to see the desire to learn and to hear her questions. This is how these people become as good as they are.

One final thing, Mike is quite happy with everything, he said to me today a few times that today is the first day, that he can see a light at the end of the tunnel. He is seeing the light we have seen all along. Today was a game changer. As our occupational therapist is in the room talking to Mike (her work is done, and now just chit chatting) I look in the hall and see 4 bodies. I got so excited, and I start waving. In the room comes Mike's 3rd floor physio girls... minus Yvonne, Yvonne. The 4 of them come in all eye smiles. These 4 women came up after their shift to see Mike. This is the extra ... this is just honestly, beyond words. They are as happy to see Mike as he is to see them. Oh, he loves these girls. He says thank you girls, you pushed me, you watched me from the first time I sat, till my last walk down your hall. These girls... forever in our hearts, my gosh... you enjoy this

Steady As We Go.

amazing success in this room. Ok this was an amazing day, banking on Mike's gout pills arriving on time, I am sure he will have a sound sleep, in a bed without a tube in his neck, with only a feeding tube left for now and an iv in his arm and monitors on his chest. The light is being seen ... the light to earthly healing and to coming home. Now it is time to rehab, to get stronger, to breathe better, to relearn skills. Today finally, I see the light today, Sarah, I am going to get there. I know you are Mikey.

Individual prayer requests:

For complete healing of Mike's body

Pray for peace of mind and confidence

Anytime someone comes to visit Mike from 3 he asks about Colton and Colton is still there so pray for Colton and for Kim whose bed was across from Mike here in step down

Pray for our world

Quotes for tonight:

"Don't limit your challenges, challenge your limits."

"Don't worry about how things are going to work out, just believe they will."

"Sometimes you can't see the light at the end of the tunnel... it's not that the light isn't there, it's that there is a curve you went through in the tunnel."

As always:

Beat the bumps Mikey

Let go and let God.

If you ain't cheatin you ain't tryin

steady as we go

Love Sarah

Scripture:

Zephaniah 3:17, The Lord your God is with you, he is mighty to save. He will take great delight in you, he will quiet you with his love, he will rejoice over you with singing.

Reflection:

I found this written in my notebook from June 8th.... Don't forget while you are busy doubting yourself, someone else is busy admiring your strength. How true is that! I wrote how on this day Mike could for the first time believe that he was going to at some point reach his goal of going home. I watched from his first stand the self doubt he had. The disbelief in his strength. It was never a disbelief in the physio, he knew they could do it but was unsure of his own abilities. DOUBT. But everyday he was admired by all he accomplished. That's why they fist pumped him, applauded his walks, eye smiled every time he accomplished what they asked. It's why physio visited him after work because the whole time he was busy doubting himself... they were busy admiring his

Steady As We Go.

strength of will and character. I believe that true in life. We are doubting ourselves, yet someone else is finding strength watching us do the very thing we are doubting ourselves about. Then we watch with admiration someone else do something that they are doubting they can do! We should just all believe in ourselves and put doubt aside and see the confidence in ourselves that we are so able to see in others.

Author Sarah VanNetten

THE LITTLE THINGS

Day 63/ June 9th

I am so pleased with how Mike is doing. What he could not do even 3 days ago, he has more strength now. Today will be another new day of new triumphs and hurdles met. He is truly marking a path in the medical research field. Mike is the research now for Covid and ECMO and how the long-term effects of this virus will be for survivors. I am so happy that he can be a part of this. So happy that we have this chance to help other people. Finally, Mike can be the help to others he is so used to being.

So here is what I learned today about my Mikey, your Mike, your Chicken. Mike had a good night sleep, and you will all be happy to know that the gout is under control. His foot is feeling much better. He is doing well on the real food. Appetite will take time to return but he is appreciating real food again. Mike's doctor was in this morning, and they are so pleased with how he is doing. His latest lung x-ray is a miracle in the improvement. … Of course, it is… one more miracle in the long line of miracles that he has accomplished. Mike will be a part of a couple studies that will continue here at the General. He is happy to do anything. He is just so grateful for all the people in this hospital. It is busy afternoons between doctor visits and his bed exercises. He has bands to use as well, to gain more strength and to help with flexibility. Mike is his usual kind self. He also does not suffer from headaches or nightmares or any changes to his personality. He is the same guy as before… we just must get his strength back. Mike had physio today again, back up and walking with his girls, his foot did well. Mike wants to keep

Steady As We Go.

making strides. When he arrived back to his room he asked if he could walk into the room and into his chair without the walker, and with one of his girls on either side only to walk beside him, he made it to his chair. So proud of him.

Every person we have encountered in this building I admire, while physio is walking him, they also ask about our family and kids. You learn about their lives. Today after physio Mike's room was cleaned, this too was another person. This woman loves her job and life, not because she loves cleaning rooms (she does not mind it), but because she loves people and their stories. she loves to get to know the patients as she cleans. She loves to get to know the family as she makes the room so tidy. Finds a spot for everything. She is grateful for her life. She enjoys her job but loves her homelife. She loves to sit in her hot tub and listen to the birds, she loves to hang clothes on the line. She loves the simple things in life. Before she left, she asked if she could do anything else, she knows these nurses are busy and she wants to help make their lives easier, so she gets Mike a big cup of ice and gets me a drink. Thank you for loving your job and making a difference.

Hopefully tomorrow or the next day Mike will have his feeding tube removed. Almost nothing left on his body. He is getting there; we just need to figure out the next best plan for Mike and it will be the best plan as they have not steered us wrong yet.

Thank you for your continued support and prayers. A shout out to Kansas City Brad (Kristin Turner) Brad came off ECMO today and is still sedated but Kristin is so happy...

rightfully so. So many new and helpful things are being learned about Covid. So many people are getting their second dose. Continue this great work my friends., continue praying and continue to enjoy the little things in life... they are what makes life worth living.

Individual Prayer requests:

Pray for complete healing of Mike for a return to normal life.

Found out today that a friend in Brantford Brian Windle is in hospital with some pressing concerns (not covid related). Everyone knows someone struggling... keep asking for answers, God loves to be asked

Pray for God's healing of our world and lives.

Quotes for tonight:

"God's grace is not the light at the end of the tunnel. its the light that guides us through it."

"Be patient with yourself. You are growing stronger every day. The weight of the world will become lighter... and you will begin to shine brighter. DON'T GIVE UP!"

"Don't wait until you've reached your goal to be proud of yourself. Be proud of every step you take towards reaching that goal."

As always:

Beat the bumps Mikey

Let go and let God

If you ain't cheatin you ain't tryin

Steady As We Go.

making strides. When he arrived back to his room he asked if he could walk into the room and into his chair without the walker, and with one of his girls on either side only to walk beside him, he made it to his chair. So proud of him.

Every person we have encountered in this building I admire, while physio is walking him, they also ask about our family and kids. You learn about their lives. Today after physio Mike's room was cleaned, this too was another person. This woman loves her job and life, not because she loves cleaning rooms (she does not mind it), but because she loves people and their stories. she loves to get to know the patients as she cleans. She loves to get to know the family as she makes the room so tidy. Finds a spot for everything. She is grateful for her life. She enjoys her job but loves her homelife. She loves to sit in her hot tub and listen to the birds, she loves to hang clothes on the line. She loves the simple things in life. Before she left, she asked if she could do anything else, she knows these nurses are busy and she wants to help make their lives easier, so she gets Mike a big cup of ice and gets me a drink. Thank you for loving your job and making a difference.

Hopefully tomorrow or the next day Mike will have his feeding tube removed. Almost nothing left on his body. He is getting there; we just need to figure out the next best plan for Mike and it will be the best plan as they have not steered us wrong yet.

Thank you for your continued support and prayers. A shout out to Kansas City Brad (Kristin Turner) Brad came off ECMO today and is still sedated but Kristin is so happy...

rightfully so. So many new and helpful things are being learned about Covid. So many people are getting their second dose. Continue this great work my friends., continue praying and continue to enjoy the little things in life... they are what makes life worth living.

Individual Prayer requests:

Pray for complete healing of Mike for a return to normal life.

Found out today that a friend in Brantford Brian Windle is in hospital with some pressing concerns (not covid related). Everyone knows someone struggling... keep asking for answers, God loves to be asked

Pray for God's healing of our world and lives.

Quotes for tonight:

"God's grace is not the light at the end of the tunnel. its the light that guides us through it."

"Be patient with yourself. You are growing stronger every day. The weight of the world will become lighter... and you will begin to shine brighter. DON'T GIVE UP!"

"Don't wait until you've reached your goal to be proud of yourself. Be proud of every step you take towards reaching that goal."

As always:

Beat the bumps Mikey

Let go and let God

If you ain't cheatin you ain't tryin

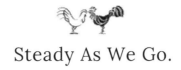

Steady As We Go.

Steady as we go

Love Sarah

Scripture:

1 Thessalonians 5:17, Pray continually.

Reflection:

　　The little things in life really are the big things. All the money in the world really can't buy health or happiness. Why does it sometimes take for bad things to happen for us to remember this? The little things are the things worth remembering. Someone said to me the other day… yep, he will be the richest person in the cemetery! I had never heard that saying before. Boy oh boy, what a thought. There is most definitely nothing wrong with money, we most definitely need it to survive but along the quest for it, I hope we all have the chance to look for the little things that bring the joy and happiness and make the memories that we have. I hope we can all have a bit of the joy I saw in the cleaning lady's life everyday she came into Mike's room. It's the little things that are truly the big things in the end.

Author Sarah VanNetten

GOOD DAYS

Day 64/June 10th

During this time, I have written many things. Some were written in the heat of the moment, some in complete fear, panic, begging. Some in hope, in joy, in admiration, in wonder and awe. The number of different emotions I have felt during this time... that we all have felt during this time is overwhelming. Now Mike is experiencing these feelings too. He is overwhelmed with gratitude. He is emotional with thanks. Today I read that ... "How you are, is not who you are," I got thinking about this, and it rings true. How we are, physically, emotionally, defeated, tired... it is not who we are. Who we are, is something we choose from the inside-out. Who we are, comes from the roots of our being, our strength, and our faith. You look at the Humboldt survivor who we see has now stood for the first time since the accident. How he was, it did not define who he is or what he will accomplish. The image that we all have of ourselves, we can change it... to better it. A daily goal to make our own image one that can make other people feel better about themselves. Several times a day, Mike says to me and anyone in the room... this is a good day. Yes Mike, today is a good day.

So here is what I learned today about my Mikey, your Mike, your Chicken. Mike continues to do well. He is an easy patient for them. He just wants to please his nurses and his doctors. Mike had some physio this morning and we are now ready for shoes. He has his own wheelchair, walker, and oxygen tank... the room is full! The days are surprisingly busy with the pop ins and meetings. Mike needs to start spending more time in his chair. He needs to eat all meals in his chair,

Steady As We Go.

be doing his exercises on his own and walking with his physio in afternoon. He can get himself from bed to chair if someone is there. This morning Mike walked to the bathroom with his nurse to brush his teeth. It is the first time he has seen himself in a mirror and he was shocked... he looks fantastically alive and beautiful, but his arms are skinny, as are his legs... his legs he has looked down and seen, but not his arms! All this can be regained! He knows this, and he will! Another big feat was that today the feeding tube was removed from his nose. What a relief! Only an IV left in and monitors on his stomach. We are getting there. A 'good day' Mike says! As supper arrives two visitors pop in, Miranda and Yvonne! Physio girls from 3 just to pop in on their own time to visit and see his progress. What a great visit! They are amazed at how much stronger his voice is. He sure enjoys talking to these girls. He said to them, (physio was always at 2). I used to watch the clock and dread 2 o'clock. I hated it, but then I started getting stronger, I watched the clock and started waiting for 2 o' clock (keep in mind this was not an overnight love). The love Mike has for all that was done for him on the 3rd floor continues. Rehab is important for Mike and those decisions are being made now. We want the most thorough rehab. We want to finish this process. Mike is so wanting to be home, but he never wants to come back through these doors as a patient... he wants to come back through these doors in the swagger he had before with the smile they are beginning to know and the sparkle in his eyes. He will come back through as a survivor and a miracle.

Prayer requests for today:

Pray for 8th floor medicine... a new different busy that has so many different types of illnesses they are dealing with all the time

Pray for a complete healing of Mike, body, mind, and strength

Pray that as we enter phase 1 people are kind!

Quotes for today:

"Always remember, your focus determines your reality."

"Our wounds are often the openings into the best and most beautiful part."

"Do everything with a good heart and expect nothing in return."

"Change is not a bolt of lightning that arrives with a zap. It is a bridge-built brick by brick, everyday, with sweat and humility and slips. It is hard work, and slow work, but it can be thrilling to watch it take shape."

As always:

Beat the bumps Mikey

Let go and let God.

If you ain't cheatin you ain't tryin

Steady as we go

Love Sarah.

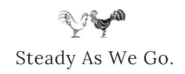

Steady As We Go.

Scripture:

Luke 1:37, For nothing is impossible with God

Reflection:

Give your mind a break from planning and trying to anticipate what will happen. This morning I am sitting on a deck in front of a glass like lake, watching a paddle boarder glide across the water with not a ripple in it. It is a good place to give your mind a rest. These devotionals I have read during this time of my life have been just what the doctor (or God) ordered. Our brains (or at least mine) get so busy with planning and anticipating what is going to happen next to try to plan for the circumstances we are not even sure will happen. It's constant for some from the moment they wake up till bed and sometimes during those hours too. This morning as I look out at the water and the paddle boarder, I wonder what is going through their head… probably not much I hope other than the calming stroke of the paddle through the water. Sometimes we just need rest, a mind break, asking for help through prayer for the day to be taken care of for us.

BEAUTIFUL DAYS

Day 65/ June 11th

A friend who texts me every morning started it out like this today. 'Good morning! Well, this is getting repetitive-but it's another beautiful day!' My response to her was that good days are never repetitive...Good days should be cherished and stored away for days when the sun and the light are a little harder to see. Beautiful days can never get boring or old. I hope our world is at the start of seeing so many consecutive beautiful days in a row. Days of hope and light and love with kindness and friendship, filled with smiles and tears of joy. I hope we all hold more appreciation for blessings we all have. Cherish them.

So here is what I learned today about my Mikey, your Mike, your Chicken. Mike is sleeping at night far better without so much equipment on his body. He only has the 'stickers' on his chest and stomach to monitor his oxygen and his heart rate as well as an IV site in his arm for antibiotics. He looks better every day. He is now used to floor 8 and the comings and goings of it. Nurses take care of more than 1 patient up here but are always kind and take the time to inquire about all issues and to even learn about their patient and their lives. We had another busy day. After lunch in his chair, he did some of his exercises with his stationary foot pedal machine. We went for a wheelchair walk around the ward for a while. Then it was time for physio today. Beth has worked with Mike several times now and they have a good understanding of each other. Mike's 'the gout' foot is feeling so much better. It does not affect his walk, so he got a good

Steady As We Go.

long one in with his walker. His pace is quicker, his form is better, his confidence is so much stronger. When he rests his recovery is better. He can talk again quicker. He can say, let's go again. We do a lap and a half of the ward. These people are now also getting to know Mike... he says hello to one man wiping down a bed, then looks at me and says, "He has moved my rooms before." Finally, he is starting to remember some of these amazing people that have helped him. Back in the room he sits in his wheelchair for a bit.

      We know that Mike's next step is rehab. That has been the debate, what is the best option for him? Where should he go? I am beyond thrilled to say that today we found out that Mike will remain here in Hamilton, directly next door and attached to the General at The Regional Rehabilitation Centre and will start rehab next week! We could not have gotten better news. It is what we have wanted and what we have advocated for. For various reasons, we were unsure if it would be a possibility, but it is. The General has become a special place for Mike and me. For now, a second home... an amazing home, full of what for now... and truthfully always will feel is our family. I will forever be grateful to the Norfolk General and Burlington for their quick care and assessment of Mike to keep him moving along on April the 10th he found himself flown into this building... the General. I know that the ultimate healer is God and prayer... but through both, the people within this building with their God-given skills and minds saved Mike's life, several times. Mike came in these doors, and we feel with all our hearts that it is these doors we want him to walk out of... well. This building, these people, they deserve to see completed what they started and believed in what they were doing. They deserve to keep being proud, they deserve to keep learning. The General deserves to complete this ever so important job they started. They deserve a COVID success story. Thank you to all those who advocated for this. I am so happy to start this next leg. Also thrilled that money raised from our fundraiser 'Stride for the General'... goes to my 2 most favorite causes, an ECMO machine and the rehabilitation center. We both are so happy. Thank you, team, for making this happen.

Today I was also able to wheel Mike outside on my own for some fresh air and just to sit and watch the comings and goings around. He has had a busy day. I think he should sleep well. After supper, he is in bed waiting for the Jays to start.

I am thankful... a thankful that words will never express... what these days have been, what the support has meant, the private messages of people's stories, the comments on Facebook, the shares, the knowing how maybe Mike's story has helped you. I would have never guessed but anyway, that is for a post in a few days. I always promised myself I would carry these posts through to (at first, I said trach removal) but I have changed it to rehab start. I am spending longer days at the hospital now, a good half the day. When rehab starts, my focus will be on Mike and our kids, a balance as best possible. I want Mike home as quick as he can safely do it... he does too. Know that he will be in the best of hands, and I will still update, but just not every night. I know he is still your Mike and your Chicken. But let us not count our chickens before they are hatched. We have a whole weekend of work ahead of us yet! Steady as we Go.

Individual Prayer Requests:

For complete physical healing of Mike from Covid effects

Steady As We Go.

For the continued first and second vaccinations of our province and country

For these doctors, nurses, RT, PT, perfusionists, X-ray techs... and on and on within these buildings

Quotes for tonight:

"Life can only be understood backwards; but it must be lived forwards."

"Don't forget while you are busy doubting yourself, someone else is busy admiring your strength."

"Not all storms come to disrupt your life, some come to clear your path."

As always:

Beat the bumps Mikey

Let go and let God.

If you ain't cheatin you ain't tryin

Steady as we go.

Love Sarah

Scripture:

Colossians 3:23, Whatever you do, work at it with your heart, as working for the Lord, not for men.

Reflection:

Although it truly was not that long ago, I remember so clearly being told that Mike would be able to stay in Hamilton for rehab and just the relief it brought. Once again something that we had prayed for and was answered. I read recently, do not let fear dissipate your energy. How true! Fear can take every bit of energy you have and leave you laying in a heap on the ground. I know of many people still living in this fear for many reasons … but I know of those whose loved ones are suffering still from Covid. Their battle continues, the doctors and nurses still work hard. I hope so many of them can follow in Mike's steps and to be able to move from wing to wing and then to rehab. It is a long process, there is no denying that but a path that I very much want everyone on. That fear … it's a monster. Don't see it as a weakness. It's a vessel, pray through it, rise above it, become fierce against it.

Steady As We Go.

PURPOSE

Day 66/June 12th

Purpose, my friend Ann today sent me one last devotion. It's title was purpose. How appropriate it was for her ending devotion to me. By far not the end of her advice, or friendship, but she is a prayer warrior, and many people need her help. Move on warrior Ann! So here is what I have learned about purpose. It is the reason why something is done or used... The aim or intention of something... the feeling of being determined to do or to achieve something... the goal of a person. Did my purpose ever change on April 8? It was a gradual change, I guess I suddenly had a purpose in life maybe... I had always had a purpose to be happy, to raise good kids, to pay off debt, to have my kids do well in school and hockey, but suddenly I truly had a purpose. My purpose became Mike. My purpose became how to keep Mike alive. My purpose and existence were centered in this.

I do think my purpose had some accomplishments. The purpose has turned hurts into healings for others. My main goal was to turn Mike's hurt and illness into healing, but I feel that through this, other people have experienced healing and peace for their situations.

They have been made better through this community of a friendship we now have. I have wanted to cultivate awe and gratitude. Awe for both what this virus can do to a body... but more importantly, awe and gratitude for the people we must conquer and battle this. I hope that by my posts, every single person is in awe and gratitude to both the power of prayer and absolute love and passion, these workers have for their position and their patients.

My purpose was to find and build community. Well, I found what community is truly all about. I found out what small town community is, but also what this larger community that is much bigger from a common topic which is Mike. Mike is a journey anyone could find themselves in. He would never want anyone to step foot in these shoes. The community has been built around his story. The gratitude, the blessings realized, the joy paid forward …that is purpose.

Finally, the purpose was that his story be told. Mike's story, the story that I needed to be told, so he would be kept top of mind… that was my purpose. The more people know, think, pray about Mike… the more who know about Covid, the more awareness… the better.

So here is what I learned about my Mikey, your Mike, your Chicken today. Stronger every day. When I arrived, Mike is listening to music on his phone. Might I add, damn I hate his music, after signing to him all those days, to now hear "Oh Jean," I still cringe. He is in good spirits. He has had his last monitor removed from his body except for IV. Today we spent, Face Timing with friends. He wore a t-shirt for the first time in 66 days. He is so looking forward to rehab. Tomorrow is Sunday, God's Day, a good Sunday, here is to a beautiful week.

Individual prayer requests:

For complete healing for Mike

For complete healing of our world

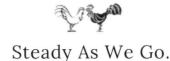

Steady As We Go.

For purpose in everyone's lives

Quotes for tonight

"The trials and tribulations in your life do not build character. They reveal it."

"Some of your greatest victories will come after your most painful experiences. Be patient, trust the process."

"If you want to find your purpose in life, find your wounds."

As always:

Beat the bumps Mikey

Let go and let God

If you ain't cheatin you ain't tryin

Steady as we go

Love Sarah

Scripture:

Exodus 9:16, But I have raised you up for this very purpose, that I might show you my power and that my name might be proclaimed in all the earth.

Reflection:

I remember writing this day and how as I was reading Ann's devotion to me about purpose it made so much sense. She sent so many wonderful words of advice and hope to me over the days of Mike. I know that someone else is benefitting from her perhaps this morning while reading what she has sent to them.

My purpose is still Mike. Although he is quite independent and quite capable, he falls high into my purpose category. All the same things do really. Awareness, health care acknowledgement, vaccines, prayer. I still want others to learn from our story. I want people who watch a loved one suffer to never give up hope. I want the recovering patient who is wondering if they can do it to read about Mike and say, yes, I can. I want for the purpose that I found along this journey to help others. God works good in all situations... I do know this. Sometimes just takes a close look to see them.

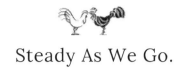

Steady As We Go.

ANOTHER CHAPTER CLOSES

Day 66/ June 13th

Today will hopefully be the last full day on floor 8 before Mike heads to rehab. Here as well we have encountered amazing care, wonderful doctors and nurses, joy in their jobs and love for making people better. While watching church this morning I once again took away a life lesson I wanted to share during these times … it was about contentment and how to choose it. A summary brought me to this conclusion. We all have our lives, but sometimes we get focused on other peoples abilities and their resources or what they have. This leads us to getting distracted and discouraged… this in turn leads us to forgetting to be grateful for what we have. Our distraction over what we don't have makes us dissatisfied… we want our neighbours car, our friends paycheck. We forget to look at what is right in front of us. We forget to be grateful for what we do have. We need to manage and love what we have. I am most definitely not saying I was always good at this, but I feel I know for sure now that money can't buy happiness… a new car couldn't give me Mikey back. I chose to be faithful that God would provide… it came with struggles and doubts and tears but always a peace that in the end that I had asked all I could and now to just continue to pray. I know now with certainty that it is not about having the most, but about making the most out of what you have been given. The 'desire to acquire', the quick hits of satisfaction will not lead to happiness. Personal relationships, love, faith … these are what lead to contentment. Deciding what is 'enough for you'. I have decided I have all I need.

So here is what I learned today about my Mikey, your Mike, your Chicken. I am writing this earlier today because I am still with Mike, and he has some things he would like to say.

"I cannot thank people enough for what support I have received. My friends, local businesses, fundraising, lights on, t shirts, chicken, decals, it's amazing…. these doctors and nurses, I can't forget about them, and I don't even remember half the things they have done for me. but I am getting a clearer picture. Physio those girls on the third floor who I used to hate and dread 2 o'clock, then actually looked forward to it. You girls were awesome. Now my new physio up here and what will be my new physio over there. I love my town and now all these people following my story … thank you. This time here …. This is not fun, it's not worth it, please get your shot, don't join my story.

I am looking forward to going to rehab, my last step before I can go home. I'm going to do it good and fast, I miss home, my family, and friends. Thank you everyone… can never repay what you have all done for me."

Mike is so true about the love and support; this is an emotional experience. Thank you for following. We had a good day otherwise up here … quiet. A FaceTime with my brother and Ang and girls… so great to see them and Byron will be home shortly for a visit and the whole fam is booked for Christmas … gotta do more things like this, live for the moment.

Steady As We Go.

I got a chance to see Mike's lung X-rays today... one from April which showed all dark, nonworking lungs, then I saw last weeks, white clear lungs, not perfect, but a medical miracle (thank you God and medicine). His Dr looked at me and said that had he not gone on ECMO, a vent would have never helped his lungs. They were too damaged. ECMO saved Mike's life ... allowing his lungs and body the time they needed to heal... I know I knew that ... but to hear it in words again... it gets me every time.

One last thing Gary and Erica brought the kids down for an outside visit. Once Mike is in rehab, he may not be having outdoor visits ... he's going to be working so a last visit until a lot of visits when he is home. So good to see them together and for Mike to finally get to see his buddies Zooey and Erica.

So here is to new adventure tomorrow, strap your new slip-on shoes on Mikey... it's work time!

Prayer requests:

For confidence in rehab and hard work.

Continue to pray for Covid patients ... may there be so many more success stories to follow in Mike's steps.

Pray for Mike's old roomie Colton. Mike asks about him all the time and he still needs prayer ... pray for anyone and everyone who needs prayer.

Quotes for tonight:

"Perhaps the butterfly is proof that you can go through a great deal of darkness yet become something beautiful."

"Inhale, exhale - all is well, all is well... all of this is part of the story you will tell."

"We get up every morning, look in the mirror and say, "Good morning fighter, today be stronger than your storm."

As always:

Beat the bumps Mikey

Let go and let God

If you ain't cheatin, you ain't tryin

Steady as we go

Love Sarah

Scripture:

Philippians 4:12, I know what it is to be in need, and I know what it is to have plenty. I have learned the secret to being content in any and every situation, whether well fed or hungry, whether living in plenty or in want.

Reflection:

The Olympics are on in Tokyo. I love watching the Olympics and all the excitement. I love all the events and the commercials surrounding the Olympics. I love hearing athletes stories and their coaches stories. What they have faced to get to where they are, their inspiration. I love the passion behind the event. These people have worked their

Steady As We Go.

whole life for a moment. A moment that might not go their way or might be the best moment of their lives. I watched the beach volleyball girls lose in heartbreak and I just watched Andre De Grasse win the 200 metre and his emotions after winning the gold. 'We all play for Canada', I love this saying. I wish we would hold it true all the time. It truly is a privilege to be a Canadian and live in this great country. We have so much to be grateful for including watching athletes and coaches proudly wearing the colours of our country and being so passionate about what they are doing and how lucky they are to have an opportunity to do this! Today's reflection I guess is more about pride, pride over seeing people reach their accomplishment, pride over people humbly accepting their defeats. Pride for hard work and effort to reach a goal. The Olympics will soon be over, but I hope our pride and that 'we all play for Canada' and unite to live as one will carry on! We truly are so blessed to have this great country to call home.

Author Sarah VanNetten

REHAB!

Day 67/ June 14th

These past 67 days I have been thinking a lot about Mike, about our lives.... All our lives, about how Covid has changed our lives, and although I firmly believe our lives will be righted it has certainly been a time of reflection. Covid is horrendous, a bastard of a virus ... I cannot say enough hateful things about it. I am trying not to hate things in life anymore... people deserve second chances and love, situations deserve forgiveness, but Covid I HATE. I hate how it has made Mike have to fight to survive and battle his way back. I hate the weakness it has put in his body. I hate how it has affected his breathing and his energy level. I hate how it has taken him from his children, his loves, and his friends I hate it with a fierce passion.

What I love is Mike. I love his attitude. I love his determination and the way he makes these nurses and doctors laugh. I love the way he thanks everyone for their help. I love the way he asks for me to pray everyday with him and asks for his love taps before I leave. I love what he is desiring and going to achieve. God is creating something new in Mike... he is really (in my opinion) a bubbling spring of joy that spills into other peoples lives, he believes in God' s power as well. Mike is going to nail this!

So, hear is what I learned today about my Mikey, your Mike, your Chicken. We made it to rehab today! Mike left another family again, floor 8 where he learned some independence and met some amazing nurses. Each of these floors is truly a family. I packed his belongings up (takes about 5 minutes) ... it's mostly the pictures peeling the tape

Steady As We Go.

off the walls … it's a well-oiled pack up). Mike is anxious and nervous but excited at the same time … it's like the morning of the first day of school… nervous butterflies. We are portered over by a great man who took Mike to his new wing. It is a beautiful new part added onto the hospital and he was greeted with love … once again they are a family … thank heaven. These people that reside in these rooms are not here for a night … they have extended stays … some long stays, they need to feel they have a new family to take care of them and feel like they have someone who cares and loves for them when their own loved ones can't be there. It is their family away from family. Everyone is kind and Mike is met by physio Michelle… Michelle who had been deployed to ICU for Covid and did rehab on Mike there is now back to her regular job in rehabilitation. Today is her first day back and Mike's first day here… so happy! This is the place we wanted to be … we are here… be content. Find contentment here. Tomorrow rehab starts, they are excited and to be honest so is Mike … he wants home in the worst way but knows it is with time. When I left, he was laying in his new bed waiting for the Jays with his water beside him and his nighttime snack readily handy (5 Oh-Henry bites and 4 m and m peanuts). "Don't worry the laying out of snacks on a Kleenex will not be lasting … I'm just still weak."

Individual prayer requests:

For confidence in Mike's heart and mind for rehab

Mike is now with stroke and spinal injuries who need prayers… all those fighting to live and accomplish feats

Pray for vaccination and for those who debate to have their hearts changed

Quotes for tonight:

"You can't go back and change the beginning, but you can start where you are and change the ending."

"New day, new beginning, new hope, new way of life. Give your best and things 'will always go alright'...." B" positive."

"I have needed God, we all do... He's God, we are not. He alone can do immeasurably more than we can ask or imagine."

As always:

Beat the bumps Mikey

Let go and let God.

If you ain't cheatin you ain't tryin

Let go and let God

Love Sarah

Scripture:

2 Corinthians 4:6, For God, who said, "Let light shine out of darkness, made his light shine in our hearts to give us the light of the knowledge of the glory of God in the face of Christ."

Steady As We Go.

Reflection:

  I still can't help it. I get so angry over Covid. I still can't believe there are people who dismiss it. I guess it mostly hurts my feelings, a bit for me and more for Mike who lived it and people would think it couldn't be, but mostly and honestly for the healthcare workers who have given up 17 months of their lives now, and some people don't even acknowledge what they have sacrificed for is real. I'm also not sure why I speak this to you... my friends, as I have never received any negative backlash... or very little. I see what is happening in the States... which is generally a precursor to us. Their cases are climbing, and hospitalization is increasing, and it is unvaccinated people. It scares me. It scares me to think that our world may go backwards again... we can't have that. My gosh I don't think we could handle that as a world. It scares me to know that those on ECMO now are unvaccinated. Yet they will receive the same love and care from these doctors and nurses because that is the oath they took. I can't imagine their inner turmoil. I can't imagine their frustration and their sadness and their pure exasperation. I can't imagine not 'getting this.' I can't imagine making posts that question what these scientists have worked so hard to figure out with a scientific background and research. I can't imagine questioning many things... someday this will be a shot that no one thinks about like the measles or polio or your vaccinations. I know we are all entitled to our own opinions... it's what makes our country free. Our country has been through a pandemic, the government did not create it. God is there to lead us through... he wants us on the other side, he gave us skills to get there... he gave us vaccines! I've seen the world through what Covid does. I have seen doctors amazement over what they can't figure out... there is an answer. Please do your part, get vaccinated, you are not immune, it could pick on you...I don't want that... not for anyone ... ever.

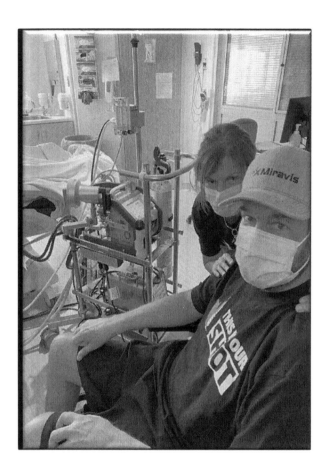

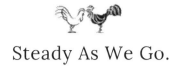

Steady As We Go.

I PROMISE TO CATCH YOU!

Day 68/ June 15th

I sit here with Mike before it is time to head home listening to one of the amazing play lists from Susan Argo Baldock-Ferguson. I think back on today. Lots of amazing things happening on this floor, not only in Mike's room but in these hallways. Mike is obviously being rehabbed for Covid and it's effects, but he is a patient in the rehab stroke unit. Another eye-opening experience and although both my dad and Mike's dad have suffered strokes and each rehabbed in hospitals, they were very lucky. Once again, I am reminded to not take our health for granted … and to not take out medical system and it's abilities for granted. Health is one of the greatest gifts we have, maybe even the greatest gift, the luxury to feel good, to walk strong, to breath deep … it's a gift. So many smiles on this floor though regardless of the challenges that they face. The song by "Mercy Me"- "Say I Won't", was posted in my comments last night. So, I listened, and I encourage everyone too. It was written by the band for a friend, Gary who in 2019 in Florida went into septic shock. He spent 107 days in hospital and left missing all 4 limbs. A verse of this song is this:

'Seeing life for the first time

Through a different lens

I'm gonna run

No, I'm gonna fly

I'm gonna know what it means to live

And not just be alive

The worlds gonna hear

Cause I'm gonna shout

And I will be dancing with when circumstances drown the music out

I can do all things through Christ, who gives me strength.

So, keep on sayin I won't

And I'll keep proving you wrong'

  This song could be so many peoples theme song up here, including Mike. From what I read Gary has 2 prosthetic arms and is awaiting his legs ... sheer determination. Count our blessings.

  Here is what I learned about my Mikey, your Mike, your Chicken today. Big day up here, Mike had his first real shower with real running water and soap since this journey began... by his smile It felt pretty good! Today was a lot of assessing, getting Mike his walker ... he is waiting on an electric wheelchair he can use to get to the gym and around, physio Michelle wants to be sure he doesn't waste his energy on getting down to the gym, but has energy to do what she wants while he is there. This should be outside his room by morn awaiting his driving instructions. Today was walking ... 3 different times and resistance testing and figuring strength level and where we want to get to. They are navigating a lot

Steady As We Go.

of ground with little research and want to have the best plan in place ... no doubt they will, all confidence is in these girls. When walks were all done for the day, we borrowed a wheelchair and went outside for awhile. They have a beautiful courtyard here, so we listened to the birds and watched the trees blow in the wind for awhile. Supper has been had... shift change soon. Thank you nurse Jackie for 2 great days. Thank you to all for your continued thoughts and love towards Mike. So many people need prayers and love around us all... so spread it around, fill your souls with peace and love and spread it out... infuse our days with positive thoughts and love and energy and watch the difference it makes.

Individual prayer requests:

For Mike, for strength, confidence, patience, and progression.

For a healing of our world

For love to beat anger

Quotes for tonight:

"Nothing in life is to be feared, it is only to be understood. Now is the time to understand more so we can fear less."

"Doing the best in this moment puts you in the best place for the next moment."

"When we strive to become better and then we are, everyone around us becomes better too."

As always:

Beat the bumps Mikey

Let go and let God

If you ain't cheatin you ain't tryin

Steady as we go

Love Sarah

Scripture:

Ecclesiastes 4:10, If one falls down, his friend can help him up. But pity the man who falls and has no one to help him up!

Reflection:

I have been thinking a lot about today's post I did, and the people Mike has had a chance to meet that are rehabbing. On the second floor Mike shared his gym and floor with spinal injuries and amputees. Now that he is an outpatient the gym is mostly shared with amputees. I have witnessed these people now for the better of two months ... the word that never comes to mind is self pity. It is such a humbling experience to be a part of this ... to push your own pity party to the side and realize, my gosh am I lucky. Their smiles, their resilience, it's amazing. Do they have their sad moments? I am sure that they do, but when it's time for the gym or hallway time, they do what my girlfriend said... they put on their big boy or girl pants and get ready to work... What a lesson. I do not know all their stories, I can only imagine, but I see their joking with each other and their physio people. The one man we see every time we are there was watching Mike do an exercise, I was standing beside him watching too... he said, "I know what is wrong with all of us who are

Steady As We Go.

missing a limb, but I always wonder the stories of the others like Mike." I quickly explained Mike's story, and the thankfulness that Mike is here to share the gym with him can make an eye leak.

There is one more thing I have learned because I asked. Third floor Physio is different, they are amazing, they promise you safety, they promise they will catch you... here in rehab it is a different land... dealing with mostly amputees... but they make the same promise, but here they will teach you how to get up. I asked physio surely people must fall here. He answered, the only promise we guarantee these people is they will fall... but we will teach you to fall safely and how to get up. Honestly, what an assurance, a bit like God, He never promised we wouldn't hit trouble or fall, but always promises if we ask, he will get us through. Like we wanted? ... maybe not but maybe something better will come from it and maybe someone will learn something from these amazing people whose glass is full. Who see the challenge in the day and go after it!?

KEEPING ON TRACK

Day 69, June 16th

What's on your mind? I still think this is the most ridiculous question. I can't think what to replace it with either, other than maybe just hey … what are you going to say. Either way, my mind is still occupied the same way, with Mike and his journey of now healing … how good. I am now more grateful than terrified. I can see an ending and coming home rather than wondering if we could keep feeling this way and not crumble. I can let tears of joy leak out instead of tears of grief and worry and sadness. I can put a smile in my eyes, and it have meaning more than trying to pretend. I will still pray, that won't end. This time has been such a whirlwind of learning. I honestly sometimes think that it was all a nightmare, but I am lucky, Mike is lucky… we all are lucky that he is just doing so well. As I have come to know, every day is a gift (for all of us) and never take anything for granted but I, my family, our friends can breathe again. For this I thank God, I truly do. The power of prayer and amazing medical staff, I will say it forever… these things saved Mike and as I live and breathe, we have all witnessed a miracle. I am just so grateful, so tonight I smile with tears of joy.

So here is what I learned today about my Mikey, your Mike, your Chicken. He had a good sleep last night! The night before he didn't. No problem, let's switch the mattress out, see how a new style works for you…much better. First full day of work. Two gym sessions and a walk today. Physio Michelle and Mike get along well together. He tells her not to keep him just because she likes him. And just because he has great

Steady As We Go.

flexibility (Mike heard that ... I missed it, I have never witnessed it). He doesn't need to stretch farther than he already has and leave better than he came in. They make each other laugh, and she makes him work. For those wondering how the electric wheelchair went. It's been busy up here today and there are new admits that need this chair far more so mike is getting a lighter weight wheelchair and can work very well with this. We got outside as well to watch the shenanigans on Barton and Victoria. It is always worth the price of admission. Sitting is becoming more tolerable too. Back to the room. Visit with staff, some friend calling, supper and time to relax for the eve. Mike is looking forward to home, me too! ... but it must be in the right time, strong enough, oxygenated enough, confident enough... both Mike and I that I can do it and take care of him. I want him safe and well. We are getting close. Patience is a virtue correct. We have followed this road this long. I trust it, God, and these medical professionals to lead to the road home.

Individual prayer requests:

For Mikes complete healing from the affects of covid to return home

For other Covid patients who are enduring this and for their families who are watching

For a hope to phase 2 and all people getting their second shot... we are getting so close

Quotes for today:

"Nothing is impossible."

"The word itself says I'm possible."

"Grateful for the small things, the big things and everything in between."

"Your mind will always believe everything you tell it. Feed it hope. Feed it truth. Feed it with love."

As always:

Beat the bumps

Let go and let God

If you ain't cheatin you ain't tryin

Steady as we go.

Love Sarah

Scripture:

2 Corinthians 4:18, So, we fix our eyes on not what is seen, but on what is unseen. For what is seen is temporary, but what is unseen is eternal.

Reflection:

I sometimes wonder why this has all happened. I think about all the people who are suffering from this horrible disease. I think, why were we so lucky when others haven't been? I know prayer has been a big factor... everyone praying for Mike and his medical teams. There is power in prayer. It helps to lighten-up even our darkest moments. I think that luck is probably not what it is about at all... but more likely a blessing from God.

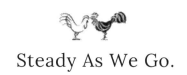
Steady As We Go.

Author Sarah VanNetten

ENTERING THE SEVENTIES

Day 70/ June 17th

From the 60' to the 70's…. And hopefully …. hopefully we don't see the 90's. That is most definitely Mike's goal and hope, and he has made it quite clear to all his friends up here. I'm writing early again. Just sitting looking out the window watching the happenings on Wellington (not nearly as entertaining as Barton) but a little calmer and more normal, and really that's what we are looking forward to in life right now. A little bit of normal.

Here is what I learned today about my Mikey, your Mike, and your Chicken. The days are busy … and routine. Breakfast is at 8, lunch 12, supper 5 and things packed in between. A workout this morning consisted of a good walker walk. When I arrived, Mike was not lying back in bed but was sitting at his little table looking out the window. Caught him up on the happenings … we are doing a small Reno at home of our bathroom … equipping it with a large walk-in shower for when Mike comes home, trying to make life easier. Lunch arrives. Starting tomorrow it will be the meals Mike picked but today yet is still just what they gave, and it was tuna salad … those that know Mike can imagine the look at the sandwich. So off to the cafeteria I went … and do you know it took me 60 plus days to learn this building has a cafeteria in the basement beyond the coffee shop in the lobby… 60 days to find out about this gem so I got Mike a western and a 'few fries.' Another afternoon workout in the gym. Can I say that both Mike and I are humbled to be here? To have the chance to watch these people rehab. Mike will walk out of here… many of these people will never 'walk' out. They are learning

Steady As We Go.

to live a new and different way, or they are learning life without a limb. Their determination is evident on their faces, their physio is so encouraging (as they have been on every floor). It is good to be humbled in your life. It is good to feel fortunate and to see the fortune in others as well.

After gym we had a great visit with a good friend in the courtyard... normal talk, not centered around illness or sickness, Mike is so sick of hearing that Covid word. It's good to feel a bit normal too. Back upstairs for a final walk with Michelle and this walk was one lap of the ward on slight oxygen and no walker ... just his own 2 feet! ... awesome, awesome work. Mike tells Michelle she might as well just send him straight home; she rolls her eyes and says not quite yet Mike ... see you tomorrow for freaky Friday.

As Mike says, 'It was a good day'. He has had supper (it met his approval) and is laying in bed. Ordered a tv today so he can watch golf this weekend ... something he loves., so that is what he is doing now. This is certainly a remarkable building, blessed that they kept Mike here. Truly blessed this whole journey for the people we have met, the awareness, and gratitude. It is said that only in the darkness can you see the stars ... and after this do, they ever twinkle bright.

Individual prayer requests:

For determined rehab to be able to come home safely

For more successes on ECMO for Covid patients

For an appreciation and a kindness of a return to more normal life

Quotes for today:

"Success is not final, failure is not fatal, it is the courage to continue that counts."

"No matter how slow you go you are still lapping everyone on the couch."

"Successful people are experts at failing. It's not the failure itself that's important, it's what you do with that failure."

As always:

Beat the bumps Mikey

Let go and let God

If you ain't cheatin, you ain't tryin

Steady as we go

Love Sarah

Scripture:

Matthew 23:12, For whoever exalts himself will be humbled, and whoever humbles himself will be exalted.

Reflection:

Life is short, live it.

Love is rare, grab it.

Anger is bad, dump it.

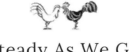

Steady As We Go.

Fear is awful, face it.

Memories are sweet, cherish them.

This was said by Winnie the Pooh! He kinda sums life up into a few words. Boy oh boy do we ever not know what life will throw at us, it could be far shorter than we ever envisioned… do the best we can with it and live!

Love is special… with that special person, it is rare. I believe there is someone out there for everyone, but when we find that person, don't take it for granted… seize it and tell it every day about how much you love.

Anger is eating… it eats you alive until there is only an empty shell, it takes your happiness away… choose against it, is what you are angry about worth it? Dump it and feel the weight leave.

Fear is awful… possibly the worst thing imaginable… all I can say is face it, use God, use prayer, use your strength which you will find inside of you… the strength you had no idea you had and face it straight on!

Memories are so sweet, make them, remember them, hold onto them, someday they will be all we have.

KEEP YOUR FOCUS

Day 71/ June 18th

The start of another weekend. A nice rain for the farmers and everyone's grass. It is always one of our favourite times to watch the crops grow. It is a beautiful time of year. Our fields are all coming up nicely and hopefully Mike will be able to take part in the fall field work... back in a tractor which he loves. Back on the farm where his heart is, and he belongs. Back to a world which is becoming more normal we hope. To a world that has hope and joy. For the longest time now, our world has not been very joyful. It is missing joy due to disease, disaster, and emotional distress. Fear and anxiety run high amidst our friends and family. Peace and calm... we must strive for. I can only pray …. that by prayer and petition and resting in our faith that our anxieties can be lessened, and we can cope better with the trials of the day! God never promised no trials or problems... but a way to cope and deal with them. It's hard to sometimes wonder why things happen or why we don't have the answers. We must trust …. This will get better.

Here is what I learned about my Mikey, your Mike, your Chicken today. Another busy day. They are good days but tiring … that's good too! Lots of hard work leads to results. Mike had his 2-1-hour sessions each in the gym and a 4 pm walk as well. He does lots of things in the gym, some arm weights, he learns how to do stairs again and is proud that he can do some without a railing. He also had to lay down on the ground and learn how to get up. He did very well. I am super proud, so was his physio, Michelle. He didn't have to

Steady As We Go.

lay there all day long. They have such a good rapport. Mike keeps asking for her to send him home and she keeps saying what would I do if you weren't here. She is so encouraging and gave Mike lots of reading material this weekend ... even though Mike was the English award winner, since that pivotal date in his life his reading efforts have declined so he will have to get his reading focus back. Life is good up here ... there is a focus. We hope not too many more weekends here. Lots of walks planned for next 2 days as no gym but still ways to get stronger. Mike (and I) love and miss all our friends ... our old ones and our new ones. Thank you for hanging in with us ... doing his best to end these posts but until then we will keep giving God, prayer and every single medical professional that chose these amazing careers the respect and admiration they are due.

Individual prayer requests:

For a world where Covid is under control and we are vaccinated

For mike to continue rehab and to prove that this can indeed be beaten

For those who suffer anxiety and worry

Quotes for tonight:

"I am not what happened to me. I am what I chose to become."

"Life is better when you cry a little, laugh a lot and are thankful for everything you've got."

"The question isn't who is going to let me; it's who is going to stop me."

As always:

Beat the bumps Mikey

Let go and let God

If you ain't cheatin you ain't tryin

Steady as we go

Love Sarah

Scripture:

Proverbs 16:9, In his heart a man plans his course, but the Lord determines his steps

Reflection:

    1.Peace and calm to strive for. 2. Anxieties to be lessened..... I mentioned these in today's post. Obviously, these things relate to me and my needs and what I was feeling with Mike, but they are something I think most, or at least a lot of struggles with. Everyday worries and concerns.

    ... Then I came across this advice. Let me help you get through this day (God). We will get through this day one way or another, the one way is to moan and groan through, while the other is to choose the path of peace and lean on God to get through. Let's face it, we have all moaned and groaned or know of someone who does, and it gets a bit much!

    We are only human, not perfect. We will struggle with finding calm and forgetting our anxieties. When this happens though... don't be upset, we have so much, going on in inside,

Steady As We Go.

pulling at us. So many outside influences. We will fail at times, let it go, slow down, be still. Know that we always have a new chance. Although today we could not find calm or perhaps our anxieties crept in, tomorrow we have a fresh start, a new start. Rest up and be ready!

Author Sarah VanNetten

GOLDEN DAYS

Day 72/June 19th

Another day almost complete, another day closer to homecoming. Another day to rest and build strength. Although we are anxious to get Mike home, we have limited control over it. He needs the time to rehab his body. He needs to regain certain functions and be sure that when he goes home, he is ready! … we only ever want to come back and visit these amazing workers to celebrate them and thank them… so we need to give others the control. I've mentioned before I have always loved having control… to have things neat and orderly and organized. I've learned though that as we all have experienced in our own lives. we lose control and then don't know what to do. I read this, this morning in my devotion, Give up striving to keep everything under control- an impossible task and a waste of precious time…. so very true. It went on to say, which is bigger, your worst problem or the God who made everything? Also, so true and such a comfort during difficult times. Finally, today I received this story from a friend Lynn Nagle and to summarize it said this …when life comes along and shakes you (which has or will happen to each of us), whatever is inside of us will come out. We must ask ourselves what is in our own cup. When life gets tricky or tough, what spills over? Is it joy, gratefulness, peace, and humility? Or is it anger, bitterness, harsh words, and reactions? Life provides the cup… we each choose how to fill it. Let there be more filling with the good things in life.

So, hear is what I learned about my Mikey, your Mike, and your Chicken today. A quiet day on the ward. It's amazing the difference on a weekend… not in a bad way it's just different. Mike and I went for several ward-walks today.

Steady As We Go.

His oxygen and heart rate are doing well with these walks. We went outside this afternoon to the courtyard to visit with friends which was wonderful. So lucky to be able to go outside and so lucky that these picnic tables can be used again. It is heartwarming to see families seeing their most loved people. Some of them for the first time. A visit can be as healing to the soul as can physio to the body. Grateful that we can do this. The late afternoon was spent watching golf and doing some Face Timing with the kids. It was a good day!

I wish everyone a nice evening, be safe, hold someone tight, be kind. May your Sunday be blessed. May your Father's Day be the best it can be. for those who have Fathers celebrate them and for those who have lost and Father's Day hurts. may your memories comfort you and bring a smile to your face. I look forward to talking tomorrow … another day closer to home.

Individual prayer requests:

That everyone up on Mike's spinal and stroke rehab floor may receive a measure of healing tonight

Pray for Father's Day tomorrow for those who will celebrate it, but more for those who will struggle with it

Pray for a world where caring dominates hate

Quotes for tonight:

"Focus on the step ahead of you, not the whole staircase."

"Don't forget to inhale-often we are focused on the exhale."

"Although the world is full of suffering, it is also full of overcoming it."

"Some people see scars, and it is wounding they remember. To me they are proof of the fact that there is healing."

As always:

Beat the bumps Mikey

Let go and let God

If you ain't cheatin you ain't tryin

Steady as we go.

Love Sarah

Scripture:

Joshua 1:5, No one will be able to stand up against you all the days of your life. As I was with Moses, so I will be with you; I will never leave you nor forsake you.

Reflection:

     For those who know our family… to say we are competitive may be a bit of an understatement … we love sports, we play a lot of them, we try very hard to be very good at them. I just finished watching the gold medal Olympic women's soccer game… Canada vs Sweden. It was on the edge of your seat; almost make you want to be sick to your stomach thrilling. It was close, it was competitive, it was gruelling. Their energy level is out of this world. Their shirts are soaked in sweat, they just keep running and running and running then run some more. Overtime with no winner and then penalty kicks, back and forth. Goalies so cool and calm

Steady As We Go.

and focused. Still no victor and now sudden death penalty kicks and within moments Canada is the winner of the Gold! … a collapse in a team pileup of pure exhilaration and joy. On the other side the emotional heartbreak of a team that was so close, but it was not the gold for them today. Different tears, different hugs, different things being whispered into their ears. My heart soared for Canada, but it couldn't help but break for Sweden as well. They worked so hard and although silver is awesome, it feels a bit … I'm sure a lot right now like a failure.

I spoke on this day about control… as much as we want total, we don't have it… impossible to get, always circumstances that come to us and change our direction. We may not ever experience the intense drive of an Olympic soccer player (they are amazing), but we all do have something we drive towards, and we all will experience intense disappointment. It was a thrill to watch this game today, to celebrate what these women have accomplished. I'd like to think that as Canadians we are humble victors as well, sympathetic to other feelings… which I think we are. The Games are wrapping up. We may never have the winning medal count but what we have is pride, love and hopefully maybe that can help unite our country and help us realize all we have.

Author Sarah VanNetten

FATHER'S DAY

Day 73/ June 20th

Father's Day today. A beautiful day of weather. A day to enjoy your dads if you still have them or spend some time remembering their importance if they are gone. I'm so very grateful beyond words that my kids still have a dad this Father's Day. I know others who battled this virus were not so lucky and so regardless of where Father's Day was this year, I am so happy to have it. Fathers (and Mothers) are more than those who created you... many people step into the shoes of moms and dads. These past 73 days. I have not 'parented' alone. I have had community by my side. I have had the most amazing friends and family 'parent and guide' so that I could be and still can be where I need to be, with Mike. Although no one can ever fill Mike's shoes... friends did help fill the role, to make sure I didn't miss anything, Zack was online for not missing anything for university in the fall, Ryan was ok in the barn, Alexis was balancing between work and school and that Holly was getting ready for grade 8 graduation. however, that should look. I know you all ask for nothing in return, but you all truly held me up and together when I was unsure I could. Bit emotional tonight ... a happy emotional ... sometimes I just think about how truly blessed we have been, how I have been a part of seeing a miracle unfold.

Mike asked me today if I ever thought he wasn't going to make it... hmmm ... how to answer. I said that I never once stopped believing in him, but doubt has a way of creeping in and with doubt comes fear and with fear panic. I never stopped believing in you Mike, or God or your teams... you

Steady As We Go.

just needed to start believing a bit in yourself... I couldn't be happier that you did. PATIENCE...involves awaiting God's time without worrying, complaining, or demanding that God satisfy our own timetable, he has his own in mind. The scripture says, "by prayer and petition for everything pray."

Here is what I learned today about my Mikey, your Mike, and your Chicken. Another good day over here on Wellington Street. We walked the ward 2 times today and increased our laps from 2-3 for both walks. Very proud of his determination. Had 2 specials visits in the courtyard today. Woody and Chal brought the kids down for Father's Day. I ordered Swiss Chalet from skip the dishes... this city living comes with its perks ... right to the front door of rehab. Don't have these luxuries in Norfolk (well other than having our cheers liquor and wine box delivered at the beginning of month, that's important too!) We had lunch together, smiles and laughs and a hope that we can do this at home soon. Thank you kids and Woods.

In the afternoon Mike's dad stopped in the courtyard for a visit too. Jack is looking good. We all look better each day Mike looks better. Another nice visit and a see you soon.

A good day... all we can ask for .... So happy Father's Day to everyone who plays the role of father but especially to our 2 Jack's and to Mike ... thank you for fighting.

Individual prayer requests:

For a good week ahead with more vaccinations, more calmness continued these covid floors.

For mike and all these patients in rehab to work hard and reach their goals… maybe even pass them."

For continued upraising of healthcare workers.

Quotes for tonight:

"Every child should remember one day that his child should follow his example, not his advice."

"Time is like a river. You cannot touch the same water twice because the flow that has passed will never pass again. Enjoy every moment of your life."

"The best is yet to come!"

"Mirror, mirror on the wall, I'll always get up after I fall. And whether I run, walk, or must crawl. I'll set my goals and achieve them all."

As always:

Beat the bumps Mikey

Let go and let God

If you ain't cheatin you ain't tryin

Steady as we go.

Love Sarah

Scripture:

Psalm20:7, Some trust in chariots and some in horses, but we trust in the name of the Lord our God.

Steady As We Go.

Reflection:

I must say, I have enjoyed reading again all the quotes... I love them. It is often hard to read the daily posts and to remember that day and what happened. It takes me right back. I am so happy that I did what I did and wrote about everyday. If I hadn't, what a blur it would now be, it would have happened, but I'm not sure to what remembrance other than a gigantic nightmare. I think it's important to never forget, for Mike to know. To read it again takes me right back to the feelings, the vividness, also the amazement and the pride. It is a journey going through these emotions again.

Yesterday post had a quote about scars and that for some they only see the wounding, but others look, and they see the healing. I love this one! It is true for when I see Mike's few scars, but I don't know any of us who don't have any scar whether it be internal or external. I can say I think I am carrying around a few internal scars from this past year. Some days I do better with them than others, but I'm going to get them ... I'm leaning on God to help me; I don't think I could without him.

Be aware of who we see around us, not every body scar is on their outside visible. Some people carry them in their heart or their mind. No one is truly capable of judging another without walking a mile in their shoes, and then maybe that's not even enough. Every scar inside or outside does indeed tell of a wound... a story. May the true story be not the wounding it shows... but the healing and the strength gained from it.

Author Sarah VanNetten

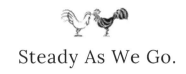

Steady As We Go.

FIND YOUR CONTENTMENT

Day 74/ June 21st

  Back to work today in the gym. The work needed so that Mike can come home. I know I have spoken before about contentment...a state of happiness and satisfaction, but the longer we are in the hospital, the more important I think it is. Right now, there is no point in chasing other dreams, envying the people who sleep in their own beds, get to go to work everyday, go to the lake, or sit on a patio. Finding contentment in where we are right now is so important to continued healing. Looking at comparisons between situations is the thief of your joy. It is often hard to compare and to be content at the same time ... for anyone. I guess this leaves us with truly being and choosing contentment (happiness and satisfaction). To strive for more is not wrong (Mike is striving for more everyday), but he must find happiness in the day as well ... we all do, to find the drive to get to the next day. We are never going to be measured by how much we own. In the end ... it's how we lived our lives that matters.

  So here is what I learned today about my Mikey, your Mike, your Chicken. He had a busy day in the gym. When I arrived at 11, he was resting in bed, his legs were tired, it was leg day. The morning had lots and lots of leg exercises. Monitoring between the exercises, oxygen and heart rate is the battle. Back to the gym at 1 for more legs ... this included a staircase, up one flight and back down. Not an easy feat. Michelle brought him back to the room and they are both so pleased. "I think my next walk should be home Michelle." ...... "So, you keep telling me Mike, but I'm not done with you yet."

Mike is just supposed to rest until his 4 pm walk so we watched a movie. I honestly can't think of the last time we did that, but we watched RV with Robin Williams and it was hilarious. Laugh out loud funny. It feels so good to laugh and to see Mike laugh and smile.

4 pm rolls around and it's walk time. Only one lap today, lots of work today... that's good enough, see you in the morning Mike. After this, before supper I took Mike for a spin around the courtyard. While we were out there the helicopter took off. We both just stood there in amazement and watched it. Mike says, "I can't believe I was in there and I can't believe I can't remember it at all." We are just so lucky... blessed to live somewhere where this is available to us. The things we take for granted. I am so grateful that Mike was able to ride in that helicopter ... it was valuable moments saved... grateful and so thankful... content.

Mike is tuckered after today, so he is resting in bed talking on the phone catching up on life and telling people how hard this work out stuff is. Love him for doing this, it's all going to be so worth it. The quotes tonight are gym quotes, motivation for workouts and success. Have a great night, friends and we will talk tomorrow...

Individual prayer requests:

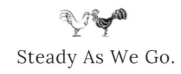

Steady As We Go.

For continued healing and rehab for Mike

Continued vaccinations … yeah!!!

For brighter days ahead … I can see them coming

Prayer for what wonderful healthcare we have

Quotes for tonight:

"The only person you need to be better than is the person you were yesterday."

"Don't stop when you're tired, stop when you're done."

"Clear your mind of can't."

"The comeback is always stronger than the setback."

As always:

Best the bumps Mikey

Let go and let God

If you ain't cheatin you ain't tryin

Steady as we go.

Love Sarah

Scripture:

Matthew 14:31,Immediately Jesus reached out his hand and caught him. "You of little faith," he said, "why did you doubt?"

Reflection:

My devotion for this day was about thanking God for what troubles you.... What? ... I think these are the struggles that nonbelievers have with believing. God wants thanks for troubles. What God asks for that? Truthfully, I have struggles even understanding this.

This is what I take from this... for me at least. I feel I am pretty good at thanking God for the good. I often acknowledge him in a sunset or down. I see him in little ways every day. I say my prayers at night. I think about him often. But my troubles lately... I am talking nonstop to God. I would never say that I know my bible well. I love my bible, the feel of it comforts me, but I don't know it like many people I know do. I do know it's comfort. My troubles, I took to God. My troubles I also couldn't understand. I spent time between asking God why and thanking God for every single improvement Mike had. It's true! You can't curse God and thank him at the same time. Troubles, we can't get away from them, how could we possibly blame God for every single one? Do we give him credit for every single glory? What does that show of our strength? I think it's our troubles that ultimately show our faith. Give God the glory, if God brought you to it, he would help you find the way through it. Let Go... Believe.

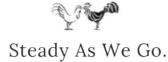

Steady As We Go.

Fight the Good Fight

Day 78/ June 25th

I'm sitting at my little corner listening to Mike and a new friend (another patient on the floor) chit chatting in Mike's room. Another conversation I never thought I would be a part of ... like 2 hens in a hen house just chattering up a storm about their gym routines, what their workout program is like, who is your physio girl. They talked about their nurses and the food. Mike, I think will be happy if he never eats mashed potatoes again. They are laughing, sharing stories. Making a normal moment out of a non normal situation. It's nice to see them laugh about things only patients would find funny.

During this time, I have received so many private messages or letters from people who tell me their story or what Mike's story has meant to them. What hearing this reality has done to their way of thinking. It's touching, some of them are heartbreaking, most are life changing stories. My intention at the start was never this ... it was only to keep my original friends and family updated on my most important situation. I had no idea what it would become and the snowball it would turn into. I am honoured and truly humbled that in any way I /we have been able to help other people. I have always felt that Mike was the only person I knew who was strong enough to endure this, to raise the Covid awareness he did, to increase the desire to be vaccinated, to be a testimony to the power of prayer and to advocate for these amazing workers that walk within this building. Strong enough to accomplish this and to come out on the living side. Many others will survive this... I do not doubt and in fact I know from the many messages I receive, but I am honoured that Mike's journey has accomplished so much good.

So here is what I learned about my Mikey, your Mike, and your Chicken today. Another truly jam-packed day. Morning workout focused more on his walking and controlling oxygen and monitoring levels. Also did stretching ... not many in that gym are big fans of the stretching factor. When I arrived, he had just returned from the gym and was resting up. Had some lunch and back at er. Afternoon workout focused on the six-minute walk without walker or oxygen. I am the timer, Renata is the monitor, he is improving all the time. Next Michelle takes him outside, with walker and oxygen and they work on walking on grass, over stones, up a ramp. They always have quite the conversation together ... what can I do to prove to you to send me home yet Michelle? A few more things Mike soon enough.

The rest of the afternoon was spent on body mass testing and breathing tests. It didn't take long for the 4 pm walk to roll around and back to the gym for stairs. Once using railings, once without. Mikey is doing just so amazing... it's wonderful to see... but what is also wonderful is to watch other people in their therapy. While Mike was recovering his heart rate, I watched a woman with the help of Michelle and Suzanne learn how to do one step from her wheelchair to her walker and up one step. These girls guidance, their knowledge, their encouragement. Another whole world of smart. She did it... she did the step, and I was just so dam proud of this woman I don't even know. As I have said there

Steady As We Go.

are no pity parties up here, there is no time. There is work to be done and a great team to get you there.

Mike was also lucky enough to get his first shot today. He was more than happy to have one more needle stick in his body for this. Never want anyone to experience his story.

Finally (lastly, I promise) when we returned to the room there was a FedEx box on the desk, it was from the Los Angeles Kings. Inside was a jersey signed by their assistant Drew Doughty. Sent with a very beautiful letter from Rob Blake and Nelson Emerson. You can never take the small-town pride out of a small-town person. Thank you so much Rob and Nelson and Drew…. Another great act of kindness in a world that needs to see light. With that once again have a nice night, enjoy your family, your pets if that is your family, your health or your strive for health. Keep going to what it is you are reaching for. As I end Mike is lying in bed listening to keep fighting the good fight. Exactly what we all must do!

Individual prayer requests:

For Kansas City Brad (Kristin Turner) keep fighting Brad

For a little 2-year-old girl Claire from Mitchell Ontario who is battling leukemia.

For Colton who is showing improved signs

Always for Mike

Quotes for tonight:

"You never lose you either win or learn."

"Anxiety does not empty tomorrow of its sorrows, but only empties today of its strength."

"Push your limits and get comfortable being uncomfortable. It reminds us that we are living."

As always:

Beat the bumps Mikey

Let go and let God

If you ain't cheatin you ain't tryin

Steady as we go.

Love Sarah

Scripture:

Jeremiah 31:3, The Lord appeared to us in the past saying: "I have loved you with an everlasting love; I have drawn you with loving - kindness."

Reflection:

  Life humbles you as you age... it makes you realize how much time you have wasted on nonsense. This quote showed up in my Facebook feed the other day. It really resonated with me. It has hit home after this past half a year. I don't think anyone has had an easy time, some just a bit tougher, but everyone with a story. I think I used the word humble so many times in my posts.

  Humble...not proud or haughty, not arrogant, or assertive.

Steady As We Go.

If as we grow older, we see all the greatness we have around us, how can we help but be humbled. I think it is something we only get as we age... the same as people say they are happier in their 30's than 20's. Then happier in their 40's than 30's. We realize how unimportant some things really were. We got ourselves worked up over that problem in our life. It's like a good bottle of wine, life really does get sweeter with time. If only we had realized this when we were young (probably would have taken away some of the fun) but it is a true lesson now. As we head forward into time, age, life... don't waste it on the nonsense of the world, whether it be people, opinions, or expectations. Seize the day, be humble in it, everyday is a gift. Celebrate it.

ADVERSITY

Day 79/ June 26th

Quiet weekend day up here. Rainy morning everywhere, I think. Greening up the grass, watering the plants and feeding the fields ... all important things. ... so, for my little lesson today I will share the following as food for thought. One of Mike's school friends sent him a link to a lesson on adversity and I thought I would quickly share what I learned. Really, we can all learn something each day. As we all know we are living in a world of disruption (this I knew even before Mike got sick). Times are uncertain, the world is a trying place now, unsure, sad, scary. Certain circumstances that we face that are so difficult are called adversity. I don't think I have ever really faced adversity before, not in the way I have through this ... but what I never considered is this. God saves THROUGH adversity, not just FROM adversity. I never considered this. Some people (Mike) must go through things, not everyone can be kept from it ... why was Mike chosen to go through it? I will never know but I have a couple of ideas. Adversity sucks, it's hard, but for those who have followed Mike's journey, they couldn't help but hear about God, what I had to say about him, my belief, my relationship. For some this might be the only God you hear about... so if through Mike you have learned to talk to God than that is a win. God can bring praise for himself through the least expected people. Through this adversity many people have changed their tune on being vaccinated again, so good. Unfortunately for God's reasons unknown to all, we can't run from adversity ... we are slammed into the middle of it. I pray for everyone caught in it that you use God to get through it, you can find a good in it, and you can share from it (lesson done).

Steady As We Go.

Here is what today I learned my Mikey, your Mike, your Chicken. He's in good spirits truly he is. Mike has made friends. His neighbour in the room next door plays her music and sings out loud quite an arrangement and entertaining ... I think she and I could have quite a gig. We did just relaxing things today... hung out so to say. Walked the ward, did 2 outdoor trips, and watched a movie recommended by nurse Joey called, 'The Choice' quite a hospital choice but very good. It's good to rest just as it's good to work. Hoping for a great day again tomorrow and a work week ready for Monday. Hoping everyone enjoys their night and their Sunday. Count your blessings.

Individual prayer requests:

For continued vaccinations

For continued rehab for this rehabilitation centre

Continued prayers for the medical field

Quotes for today:

"Sometimes when you think you are in a dark place you think you've been buried; but you have just been planted."

"Some people try to turn back their odometer-not me. I want people to know why I look this way. I have travelled a long way and some of the roads weren't paved."

"Life is not a matter of holding good cards, but sometimes playing a poor hand well."

As always:

Beat the bumps Mikey

Let go and let God

If you Ain't cheatin you ain't tryin

Steady as we go

Love Sarah

Scripture:

Genesis 28:15,I am with you and will watch over you wherever you go, and I will bring you back to this land. I will not leave you until I have done what I have promised you.

Reflection:

It has been amazing to have Mike home. To have his laundry in the hamper again, to make 2 sides of the bed, not just one, to just see him. People will ask him if anything has changed in how he is. Really not much has in his personality. If anything, he says what he is thinking, he says I love you to the kids more often, makes a point to search them out in the house and say goodbye. He has read through all the posts now and is humbled… (there is that word again).

Mike gets stopped a lot, he gets recognized, he is getting used to it. People just want to give him their congratulations, their amazement. Sometimes he knows the person, but often he doesn't. He is starting to take it in stride. Mike means a lot to many people. They prayed for his success story and want to let him know that. As I write this reflection, I am watching him out in his tractor, just for awhile, moving it around so the grass can be cut. I am so grateful. I've said

Steady As We Go.

before where I live, in this house that Mike grew up in, I love it, but he LOVES this farm. This farm runs better and is a happier farm with Mike here. I pray we are all here for a long time to come but once again… only God knows that. He has our day, our week and our lives mapped out. It is up to us to trust his road map, his bumps, his detours. May we allow him to help us to get through this life!

Author Sarah VanNetten

WE ARE ALL IN THE SAME BOAT

Day 80, June 27th

Now 80 days in. 80 days closer to home than day 1 that is for sure. I can still remember those feelings. I never really want to forget so that I can remember how quickly life can change and how much we stood to lose and how happy I am to say day 80! Mike is close, finish line is just around the corner, until then keep the focus. We know that Mike will then become an outpatient in the rehab program here which will be another welcomed step. This whole time that Mike has been here, (since awake) I have seen him in pain, I have seen him scared but I have never heard him complain. For those that know Mike, it isn't a surprise. He has never asked 'Why me?', he has never said out loud poor me, for the most part he is what he was… content.

I learned more about contentment this morning and it reminded me of Mike and yes this comes from a religious background, but you can look at it from any persons perspective because it is a reminder of happiness. The reminder is how we look at life. Do we look at our lives with an abundance mentality, or a scarcity mentality? Do we see the world with a healthy eye, or an eye that is closed? It is each of our choices as to what our viewing will be. A world loved seeing in abundance and through a 'healthy' eye…, people see you full of light. The attitude and lifestyle that we practice on the outside, will only be believable if it is believed on our inside. I think that is why people are so attracted to Mike's story. This is who he truly is … abundantly, wide-eyed and seeing life. What he believes on the inside he projects

Steady As We Go.

out... people want to be around him. I am not saying he is like this all the time ... of course not, none of us could be, but how much better would life be if everyone could be a bit more generous and grateful with a heart that remembers the purpose behind it's actions. I thought this devotion that was for today was so appropriate for day 80 and where we are on this road, 'Rest with me awhile. You have journeyed a steep rugged path in recent days (weeks). The way ahead is shrouded with uncertainty. Look neither behind you, nor before you. Focus your attention on me (God). Trust me that I will equip you fully for whatever awaits you on your journey. I am with you'. It is so appropriate for this length into the story.

So here is what I learned today about my Mikey, your Mike, your Chicken. It was a nice day. The day passed by easily. Mike and I went for a couple of walks around the ward for exercise today. We visited with the nurses who take the time to get to know you and are also so happy to share what happens in their lives. We watched some 'who's the boss making your way in the world today takes everything you've got .... Isn't that the truth. Watched some Jays game and did some Face Timing. Alida VanHamme came down to visit, her first shift back after holidays and was great to catch up. She said soon you will be home and forget all about this place .... Alida, I don't think so, we will never forget this building. Got outside for a visit with Lance Woods and Lee Woods. At times like this Mike is just Mike and it's so great to see. Lee's daughter Kaelyn made Mike a beautiful healing bracelet with a meaning of each of the stones. So many people who care. Thank you for this.

We watched the helicopter land to bring someone in desperate need come for the help this building can give. I look at that helicopter and have no idea, male or female, young or old, what has caused them to need to be here but my heart aches, my anxiety shoots, there is someone or someone's lives who've changed as of this instant. My prayers go out for this person and their family.

Mike is back in and had turkey dinner and his fav. mashed potatoes. It was a relaxing day but a good day... seeing the glass to the top. He is chatting on the phone and preparing for Michelle tomorrow and what she has in store for him. It's a new week for us all. Every day we are all going to have choices, twists, and turns, I hope sunshine and little clouds. On my way in this morning, I heard this song. "Same Boat", by Zac Brown Band. May these words be a bit of your motto for the week ahead

We're all in the same boat,

Fishing in the same hole.

Wondering where the same time goes.

Share them beaches if you're holding

Take those shots and keep reloading

If you can't be nice

Don't say nothing at all

So, help somebody who might be struggling

Spread a little love, gotta give something back.

We're all in the same boat-fishing in the same hole

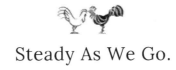

Steady As We Go.

We are all in this together my friends

Individual prayer requests:

New week, new goals for all

For all those sick and struggling both in this building and outside of it

Continued prayers for our medical professionals.

Quotes for tonight:

"If opportunity doesn't knock, build a door."

"Sooner or later those that win is those who think they can."

"Attitude is everything so pick a good one."

"Opportunity is missed by most people because it is dressed in overalls and looks like work."

As always:

Beat the bumps Mikey

Let go and let God

If you ain't cheatin you ain't tryin

Steady as we go.

Love Sarah

Scripture:

Hebrews 10:23,Let us hold unswervingly to the hope we profess, for he who promised is faithful

Reflection

If you ain't cheatin you ain't tryin. This has been Mike's saying for years. His life saying, his coaching saying, some days his mentality.

If he has ever coached your son or daughter, you yourself have probably heard this line repeated back to you at your dinner table or around the house. I'm not sure why I started including it in the bottom lines of my posts? Maybe because it reminded me of Mike, and I longed to hear his voice say it again. Mike, when he coached, was huge on effort. I loved listening to him talk to the kids. I know nothing much about hockey other than the ability to tell if my own kid had a good or a bad game. Mike had a way of explaining systems and plays to kids that made sense. He made them feel good. He made them feel important no matter than talent in the hierarchy of the team. He may tell them what they are doing wrong (it is a part of coaching) but he would always come back later with a positive. If you ain't cheatin… if your stick isn't a little before the puck, drop, if you aren't half a step offside, if you aren't a tad of a jump off the base before the pitch is thrown… you ain't tryin. Always give it, more if you can. In the end, that's what he was forced to do. A friend Chad Strohm when he shared my daily post would always add a baseball analogy to it, you didn't come to bunt, swing for the fence, get back up in the count. That's Mike, when he was against the wall, he started cheatin death and got to tryin to live. Thank you, God, for giving him the strength!

I hope one day Mike gets back behind the bench or in the dugout, he is good at it, he loves it, I think it's another of

Steady As We Go.

his things he was meant to do. For now, it is just such a treat to be able to be with him while he watches our kids play as sports start to reopen. Another wonderful gift to never take for granted!

Author Sarah VanNetten

ENJOY YOUR TUESDAY!
Day 81/ June 28th

As I sit looking out the window, we not only face the jail but also a Well-health Centre … for now a Vaccination Centre and I can sit and watch a constant flow of traffic though the one door and then back out the side door. So many different types and ages of people getting vaccinated. It is beautiful to see. During these last months, people, strangers, friends have commended me on my faith and my 'cheerleader' role and advocacy for Mike. While I am so grateful for the compliments, I can't imagine having done or having been anywhere else. A teacher from the kids grade school, Krysta Otterman a while back sent me a song to listen to called, 'Tuesdays' by Jake Scott.

"It's not just picture-perfect dancing in a white dress
It's not just rainy days where nothing stops the fighting
It is not just highs and lows and champagne toasts. I've come to know that loves not only the best days or the worst days
Love is Tuesdays." I did what I did for the Tuesdays we have had, and the Tuesdays to come. I signed up for and did the health part, but I wasn't giving up on the sickness end of the license I signed. I did what I did because I am better off together with Mike.

I did what I did because I see the same thing in him everyone does. At the same time. I know that even people who are loved are lost … why did Mike get saved, I don't know

Steady As We Go.

but am forever grateful... But I know tonight a good friend lost a friend named Troy to Covid. A 49-year-old husband and father of 2. Similar story to Mike, on ECMO but did not win his battle. My heart breaks. I know I was close to knowing that feeling and my thoughts and prayers are with this family. I pray for their comfort and for faith and friends to be able to carry them. I will never 'get' these people who think this is a hoax, what it is, is a horrible nightmare. A reality thrown at people. Honestly though that is a rant for another day and not worth taking away from today.

Here is what I learned about my Mikey, your Mike your Chicken today. Good to be back to work. The gym was alive with music, and chatter and work. All different kinds of work. Mike's consisted of arms and then 2-6 minute walks one without walker, one with. You always gain tidbits of people's lives through so much shared time. Back in the room Mike was visited by an ICU nurse that he had several times (and Alida). You may remember me talking about Stephanie and her kind calm voice. She had Mike at his worst, and she just had to come see him to give him her best and say, how excited she is to see him like this. It was nice for Mike to meet Stephanie. The afternoon workout was fun! We went outside and practiced all terrain walking. Michelle was his spotter, I was oxygen tank roller. Mike did stairs, hills, grass, rocks, flagstone, ducked under trees, I thought it was enjoyable!

Back inside for more rest, some more who's the boss and then the 4pm walk which was some stairs and ward laps. When Michelle came into the room Mike says, ' I know I am not as good as what I used to be ' and Michelle immediately said this

'I don't think that's true , you say to yourself I'm better than I was 2 weeks ago I'm not as good as I will be 2 weeks from now'... you keep your comparison into a 4 week slot, no farther ahead, no farther comparison from behind . Thank you, Michelle, words to live by, enjoy your night, see you in the morning.

There is a song I have been listening to on repeat for quite the while now ... I leave you with the chorus because if you ever play it... it is amazing!! I have sent it to Kristin Turner to listen to, and I think anyone searching for help or answers or despair can be uplifted in some way by it.

'Battle belongs' by Phil Wickham

So, when I fight, I'll fight on my knees.

With my hands lifted high

Oh God the battle belongs to you

And every fear I lay at your feet

I'll sing through the night, Oh God, the battle belongs to you.

Individual Prayer Requests:

Pray for the family of Troy who lost his battle to covid
Pray for Kansas City Brad who is being weaned from sedation, the effects on him and for Kristin to have to watch
Pray for seeing the happy in the day, enjoy the simple things

Quotes for today:

"It's what you say to yourself, about yourself, when you are by yourself...That matter most..."

Steady As We Go.

"God didn't remove the Red Sea, he parted it. Sometimes God doesn't remove your problems, he makes a way through them You know all that really matters is that the people that you love are happy and healthy. Everything else is just sprinkles on the sundae"

"When life puts you in a tough situation, don't say 'why me?' Say 'try me!"

As always:

Beat the bumps Mikey

Let go and let God

If you ain't cheatin you ain't tryin

Steady as we go

Love Sarah

Scripture....

Reflection:

To be honest, for the time being I skipped right overlooking for a scripture for today's post because I was struck by a few other things. Therefore: I need to re-read even what I wrote myself. When Mike said to Michelle I know I am not as good as I used to be... it broke my heart, but Michelle without a beat said, not as good as 2 weeks ago but better than 2 weeks from now ... how true, hopefully we all are? That one pulled at my heart strings, but it wasn't even a think about answer for Michelle...you will be better.

The second was the quote...it is what you say about yourself, when you are by yourself that matters. Do you down-talk your worth, limit your importance? Do you see your own importance, do you see your friendship values, are you a kind person? There is such a big difference between cocky and confident... not only as young adults/teenagers, but adults. God put roads in front of you... what will you let him help you with.

We all have so much potential. I hope this world works, returns to normal. None of us can see the future... I would love to, even more than before. But we can't. We can only trust and believe. Keep our faith.

(So here it is): 1 Peter5:7, Cast all his anxiety on Him because He cares for you.

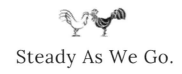
Steady As We Go.

WHAT DO YOU LOVE?
Day 82/ June 29th

W ell, I must say on hot humid days like today, it's not so bad being inside the hospital where you need your sweater on for a tad of warmth. I just have to say how as I sit and think about it… how grateful I am to be where I am now. It took the world spinning to pieces, to realize how much I have. What is important in life, what gives your life meaning, what really is happy. Can you have too much of a good thing. Going ahead will be different. A new but good different with what I hope will be an everlasting positive outlook on life. What does worry me (and it shouldn't) is that I still don't know what tomorrow brings, for anything or any of my family or friends. What awaits around the corner? Is there happiness or is there another battle to be fought. We don't know, none of us do so I tell you now my biggest challenge going forward will be to focus on the happiness and health we have TODAY. To live in the moment, to photograph them in my head (and in print). Focus and love it and not worry about tomorrow … for tomorrow has enough worries of its own, and tomorrow will take care of itself. So here is what I learned today about my Mikey, your Mike your Chicken today. Here is what I learned… that I love watching mike smile, I love hearing him laugh, I love watching him make people laugh, I love seeing the swagger that he always had when he walked back, I love to see Mike so fill of life. I still sometimes look and can't believe that he won. Rehab continues, he is doing great, working on strength, balance, oxygen, and heart. Lots of walking and lots of talking about how to handle life at home and the challenges it will bring... Michelle to Mike, "It's important that you remember that home is great, but you have to pay attention to what your body is telling you. The chickens are fine!" Yes, Michelle, you tell him.

After dinner we went outside for a visit with Mike's grade school friend Pete who also suffered Covid and was vented and came off the day before Mike went on. Both like talking, smiling, sharing a few memories and both just happy to be here. It was an awesome sight to witness 2 miracles having a conversation. Thank you, Pete for the visit. Pete says, "I can't believe it took this to get us back together, let's do it again sooner." So true, and I guess one final thought for tonight, call or text or see those people you have been thinking about, don't put it off, do it while you can and enjoy it.

Individual Prayer Requests:

For the person you pass by everyday who is sad and never even shows it.

Pray for people with anxiety about re-entering the world that they

find peace.

Pray for all those who still heal within buildings or whose hearts that grieve.

Quotes for Tonight:

Steady As We Go.

"I'm going to succeed because I am crazy enough to have believed I could."

"Being challenged in life is inevitable, being defeated is optional"

"Difficult times have helped me to understand better than before."

"How infinitely rich and beautiful life is in every way. And that so many things that one goes worrying about are of no importance whatsoever"

As Always:

Beat the bumps Mikey

Let go and let God

If you ain't cheatin you ain't tryin

Steady as we Go

Love Sarah

Scripture:
Colossians, 3:15 Let the peace of Christ rule in your hearts… and be thankful.

Reflection:

     I have tonight a bittersweet smile on my face because I read what I wrote for today… but it's difficult. Focus on today, embrace the happiness, live in the moment… dam it is hard. I haven't done the best, I'm not back to normal… I think we all know Mike isn't, that's expected. But I thought I would jump back to normal... I'm not. Why am I saying this, because I am struggling to be what is normal, to be afraid, what it is to be happy but still be able to cry on a dime. I am struggling to know that is normal.

This is one of my last reflections, I am almost done, I am always so caught up in emotion over everything. I didn't just heal. I am so awe struck at Mike, the emotions he brings out in people, I am so thankful to what we have had happen to us... more to Mike, but what happens to Mike, it happens to me. The person I have talked about, is not always me... it's the person I want to be. I have learned that healing isn't quick, Mike is going to need to nap more than I ever would have allowed, I can still be annoyed but still love, I have faith.

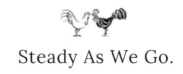

Steady As We Go.

I WANTED TO TELL YOU A SECRET
May 83/June 30th

My gosh I have not gotten through writing the date and my eyes are leaking. The words I have waited for 83 days to say... Mike is home!!!! I thought I could keep it a surprise... I forgot about media. Mike needed to set a goal and he picked July 1st... probably unachievable but a goal. As the date got closer it became obvious it was attainable. Then Mike realized that July 1st would fall on a holiday. A long, LONG, holiday and he upped his goal by a day. He did it! He is home! Nothing can stand against the power of our God!

I am going to be honest. I don't even know what to say tonight. So, tonight is not about Mike but us. We, us all. So here is what I learned about my Mikey, your Mike, your Chicken... our person, today. I am humbled to know the friends whom, I have gained through this. You know why I started this; it was for saving, you jumped aboard, people I know, people I don't and some I will never meet. I don't know why you grabbed on, but I thank you. I tell Mike, he has friends some he knew others he didn't. That you took the time to care and follow. Could we give you encouragement and hope? I hope!

But now I want to just say my thoughts and my gosh are they all over. I sit at my house desk, a different view, for sure, Mike is on his new chair that was bought for his recovery life .... My last words are for The Hamilton General Hospital. There are no words for what stands within your walls, the bravery, the resilience, the life, the love. Eighty-days ago to be honest Mike was flown to and carried within your doors and from then on you have been his home our home. You healed him, you fixed him. Physio made him, Mike again (through God's power).

Today you sent Mike off with a humbling exit. Cousin Chris Misner, you made your family, my family there will never be words. Physio girls, ECMO-man, ECMO-lady, Dr. Craig... Everyone, thank you. Thank you for everything.

Lessons for tonight because I'm not sure I can stop. Tonight, I watched a medical community celebrate Mike, I watched it, I saw people Face Timing it, I saw something that was awesome and amazing. Did I need Mike to survive? Yes, I did. But did they? Oh, my they did too! Mike is their success, their smile.

Here is what I leave you with. I do believe this has been a testimony of my faith. I do believe that by what Mike has lived and what I have spoken that even people who have actively rejected God may see his goodness.

I also ask this...for those who read this and never spoke to God... but you started praying... don't stop... keep speaking to the 'big guy'. So, someone needs your prayers because Mike needs prayers and someone else does now. Move them on.

I will never be able to end this without my heart bursting with emotion. This is it... where I wanted to be. I will

Steady As We Go.

check in during rehab but now, I need to get my family back in order. I love what each of you have invested and you each know someone in your life who needs you! So, pray that way. You have each touched me, humbled me, you have taught me as much as you say my posts have taught you. Our, stories are not finished.

Individual prayer requests:

Tonight, for Mike to adapt to being home and to being an outpatient
I pray for this 'staff', I saw the love for each other I pray for COVID to end may it soon be just a horrific memory for our world.

Quotes for today:

"It always seems impossible until It's done."

"Well done is better than well said."

"Light is giving back everything that darkness

stole."

As always:

With a few modifications: You have beaten the bumps my Mikey. Always let go and let God! If you ain't cheatin you ain't tryin! Steady as we go.

Love Sarah

PS...LIGHTS-OUT!!!

Scripture:

2 Corinthians 5:7, For we walk by faith, not by sight.

Reflection:

By faith. By faith I am here... by faith do I think I am entitled. I don't. By faith, I don't understand God's rulings or choices. Faith is a big thing. I couldn't have been able, to have been there without it.

Mike is home. He made it... I believed but am I just amazed. It comes down to faith. Faith won't heal, it won't cure, it won't promise, but it will carry you through. Faith in God.

A LITTLE NOTE, BEFORE YOU GO.

Here I am, at the very end of August, looking back... almost unbelieving. How did I get here? Not intentionally, I guess, I grew to- here. I came from a person, a home that was quite comfortable with the way lock down life was becoming. I liked being home. I liked cooking. I liked quiet nights; I loved my family. I can't pretend we lived completely by the rules.

Had we ... I wouldn't have this story, but we did our best. I thought we did great. That's the thing about Covid 19. It doesn't care. You can't convince yourself you are safe from it, or that your faith will carry you

Steady As We Go.

through. Your faith, nor that of your family will GET you through. Not every person will have the ending that we have. If you walk in my steps, I pray it gets you through the way it did for me. I guess I can't end this book without saying where I came from... from a normal life, not extravagant, not crazy, fun but normal. God as our God, to where I am now, where we are now.

Mike is a Miracle, I have said it a thousand times, I will say it a thousand more. I look at him and my jaw drops... I can never talk enough about him... but for me. How have I changed? My faith. It's stronger, there is power in prayer. Why do bad things happen to good people? Why are some saved and not others? I do not have an answer. I know the world can't be perfect because we aren't. How would you ever appreciate the beautiful sunrise without the vicious storm the night before. God is there, He was there the whole time, He's still here. I still need Him. I still talk to Him every day and pray. My mom used to say, you are never alone, you always have friend in Jesus. Yes, you do.

How have I changed? ... I don't mind hugging now... that's big! I am emotional, I can cry on a dime which is not me. I protect, I empathize and cry over countless people who send me their stories, I pray for them. I talk to God. I watch Mike get recognized and watch him do what I knew he would, secretly hate it but do anything he could to help others.

Where is my future? Loaded question! I guess honestly where God decides it to be… with Mike, I love him with my soul. But honestly after this, every day truly is a gift so the future I hope and pray for, but I must enjoy today, to laugh, to love, to have empathy. I pray that no one else will have to go through what my family went through. I will go steady as we go and try my best to let go and let God.

My gosh friends, family, medical staff, God! You were with us. From the bottom of my heart, all my love. Stay safe, stay well, and believe!

Love Sarah

A FEW PHOTOS FROM OUR JOURNEY:

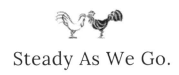

Steady As We Go.

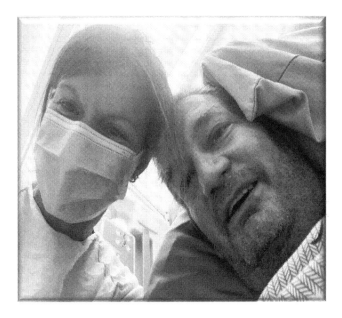

This picture is of when Mike woke up!

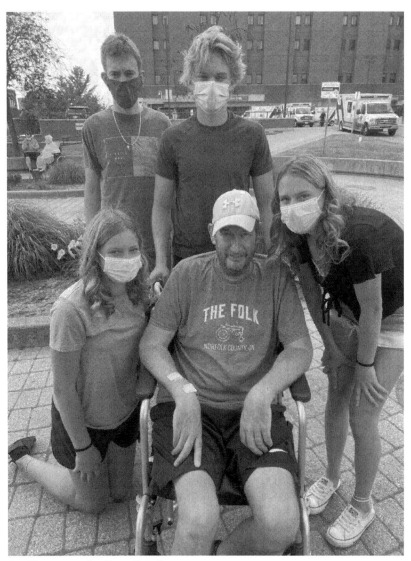

Mike and the kids.

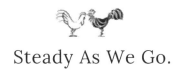

Steady As We Go.

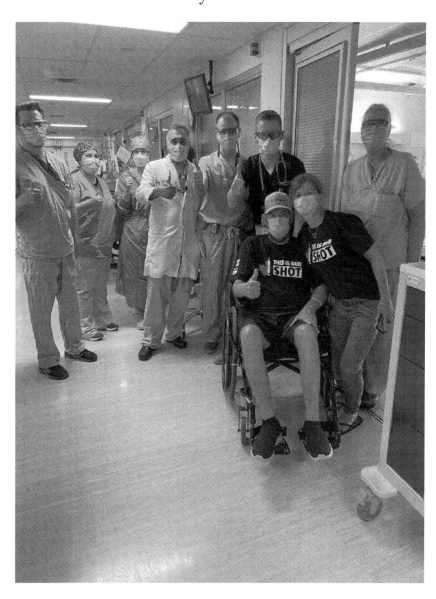

MIKE, SARAH, AND THE MED TEAM.

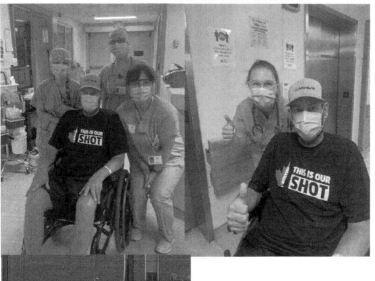
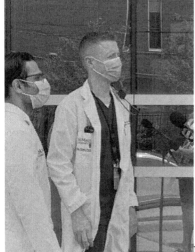

MIKE'S MEDICAL TEAM

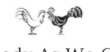

Steady As We Go.

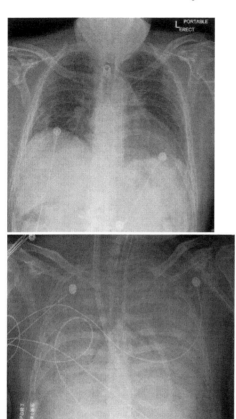

MIKE'S X-RAYS/ MIKE GRATFUL TO GET HIS SHOT!

Author Sarah VanNetten

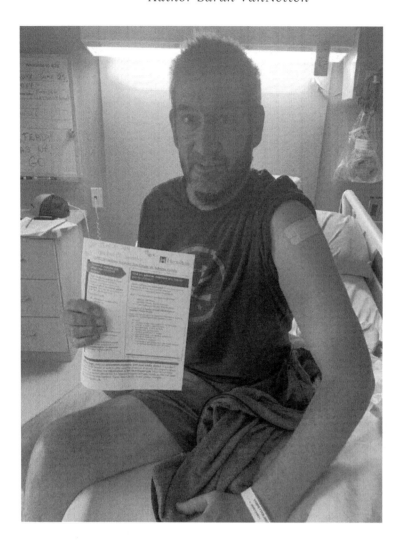

Steady As We Go.

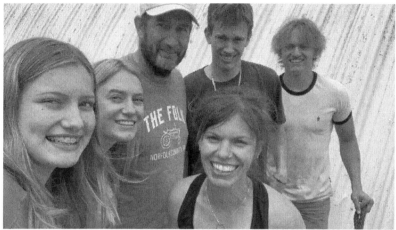

Included in photos are: Zack, Ryan, Alexis, Holly, Mike, Sarah and Denver the VanNetten family dog.

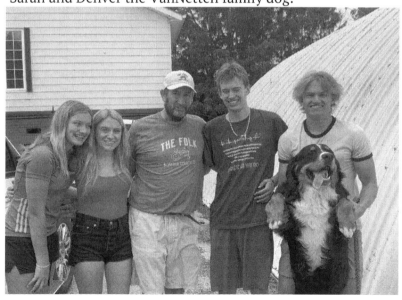

Author Sarah VanNetten